Dr. Miriam Stoppard's New
Pregnancy
& Birth Book

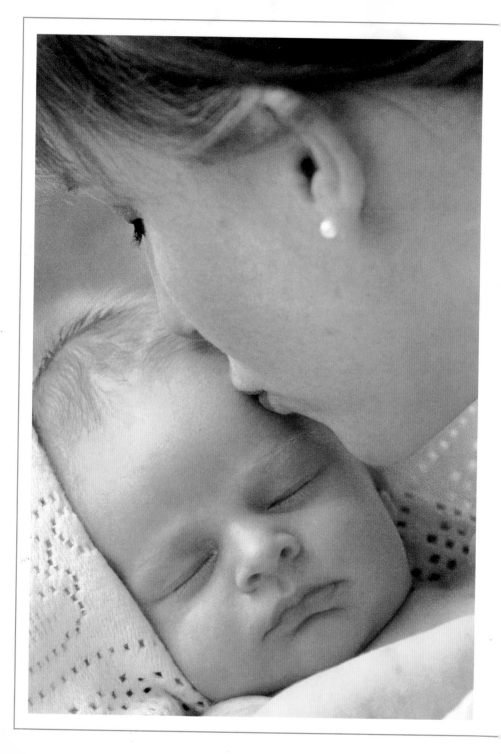

Dr. Miriam Stoppard's New Pregnancy & Birth Book

Miriam Stoppard
MD FRCP

Black-and-white photography by
Nancy Durrell McKenna

BALLANTINE BOOKS • NEW YORK

A Ballantine Book
Published by The Ballantine Publishing Group

Copyright © 1985, 1991, 1996, 1999 by Dorling Kindersley Limited, London
Text copyright © 1985, 1991, 1996, 1999 by Miriam Stoppard
Black-and-white photography © 1985, 1991, 1996, 1999 by Nancy Durrell McKenna

www.randomhouse.com/BB/

ISBN: 0-345-43795-0
Library of Congress Catalog Card Number: 99-90838

Cover design by Barbara Leff
Cover photos: (top) © Rob Lewine, (bottom) © Elizabeth Hathon; spine:
© Norbert Schafer; back cover photos (clockwise from top) © Ed Bock,
© Michael Keller, © Dimaggio / Kalish. All photos courtesy of The Stock Market.

First American Edition: January 2000

10   9   8   7   6   5   4   3   2   1

Contents

Introduction

It is a long time since I wrote my first book on pregnancy and childbirth and much has changed since then. One of the most important and welcome changes is the switch from doctor-supervised pregnancy and labor to one in which midwives play a major role. The concept of the "team" midwife is now adopted everywhere. Within this scheme of working, the prenatal and postnatal wards are mixed up together and the team of midwives on these combined wards remains the same. This ensures a unique continuity of care in which you will be seen by the same group of midwives during your prenatal care, your labor and postnatal recovery, making pregnancy and hospital birth a happier and more relaxed experience than it has been in the past. Women, midwives and doctors all benefit from this scheme. Mothers are able to become friends with the midwives in the team during their pregnancy. Care among so many skilled hands is assured, and with so many normal births, doctors are free to handle the more complicated ones that need their attention.

Technology has moved fast. Chorionic villus sampling and ultrasound scanning techniques have become so sophisticated that the majority of women who need it can benefit from the early diagnostic information they can supply. This means that a woman whose baby is at risk of inheriting a chromosomal or genetic disorder can be diagnosed within the first 10 to 12 weeks of pregnancy and, if she wishes, can opt for an early and safer termination than was possible in the past. Fetal medicine is also so advanced that in some centers a problem such as a heart defect or blood disorder can be detected and treated in the uterus, but the morality of these interventions continues to be a matter of fierce debate.

More and more information is available about maintaining the health of the pregnant woman and we are aware of the health hazards of certain food-borne diseases which can affect the fetus. Women are being warned to be meticulous about not only the food they eat, but also how they prepare it.

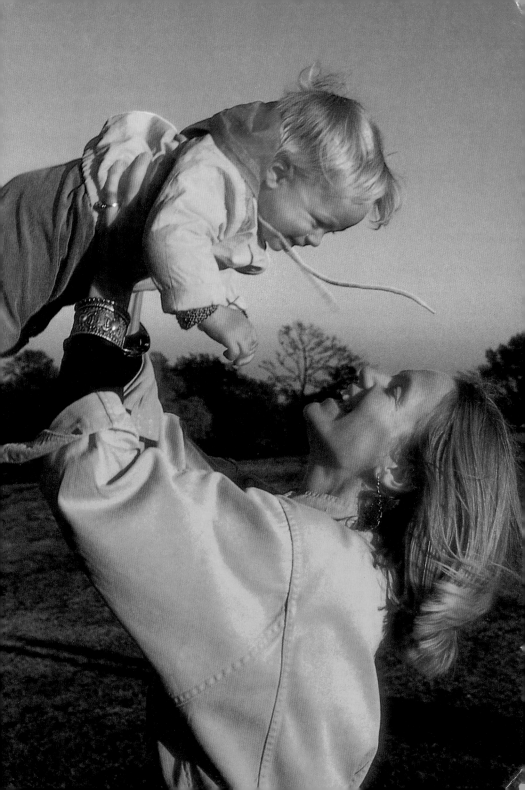

Pregnancy, labor and birth ought to be joyful experiences for a woman and her partner, and above all else I hope this book will help you both to feel really positive about pregnancy and birth. For this to happen, it is important to know what options do exist. Armed with this knowledge you will find the courage and enthusiasm to ask questions and get the information you need in order to exercise your options and make choices that suit you. It's difficult for you to discuss the pros and cons of the different medical interventions that may be suggested with a doctor or midwife if you're not familiar with the process of pregnancy and the mechanics of labor. Without some basic facts it's difficult to understand what the best positions for labor might be, for example. So this book aims to outline the options that lie before you, and then, having decided on what suits you, to give you the courage to try to get the delivery and birth you want. I have included not only useful information to help you to have a reasoned discussion with a doctor or nurse, but I have also given lists of possible questions to ask when choosing a hospital.

My other aim in writing this book is to remove fear and mystery by presenting information as openly and objectively as I can. It's been known for decades that fear of the unknown in pregnancy has a direct effect on labor and delivery; it causes pain, discomfort and slow, difficult labors. If, on the other hand, a woman has been trained during her pregnancy to listen to and observe her body, to read its messages, to act with them and help them, particularly with breathing techniques, relaxation exercises and exercises for the pelvic muscles, she can greatly assist herself in shortening the birth, making it less painful, a great deal more comfortable and a truly joyful event.

Fathers

THERE IS MUCH RESEARCH to show that if men are involved from the moment pregnancy is confirmed they become active and enthusiastic fathers. This means being involved in all the preparations, in attending prenatal classes and clinics, in decisions as to where and how to have the baby, and being involved with the care of the baby from day one. If men are shut out at any stage, the role of father is more difficult to assimilate. There is no greater help to a pregnant woman than an interested and sympathetic

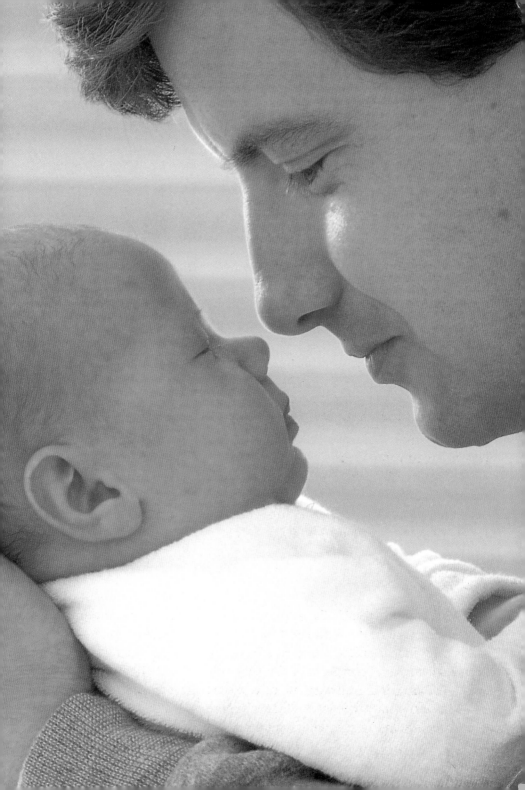

partner. There is no better medical attendant in the delivery room than an understanding, supportive father and there is certainly no better help with a newborn baby than an active, passionate dad. The labor itself can be just as remarkable an experience for the father, as this letter testifies.

❝ Regardless of where the baby is being born, at home or in the hospital, be prepared to leave your sense of embarrassment somewhere else—you will soon realize that what is happening to your wife is the most real thing she's ever experienced. She may groan and moan softly or loudly, become totally uninterested in you, ask you questions you have no answers for ("How much longer?"). So since she's putting her whole self into the labor, it will help her and you if you become as totally involved as possible. You can help her greatly by answering the questions the nurses ask and by making the decisions—she's in no state to think about anything but what is happening to her body—and above all be positive. Never cast even a shadow of doubt into her mind. Always tell her that she's doing well, because, no matter what she is doing, she's doing the best she can. Do not judge her—help her, give her some of your energy. The amount of togetherness you discover during the birth of your child will remain with you and grow for the rest of your lives. **❞**

A major priority for a pregnant woman is to have adequate help and while the best help may be a partner, it doesn't have to be. It may be more practical and even more emotionally supportive to have a close friend or relation—your mother or sister, for instance—to be your birth assistant. An option you might like to exercise is having both your partner and a friend with you during labor. To clear this path necessitates long-term planning and involvement from the beginning for all concerned with your prenatal classes, your visits to the hospital, and chats to midwives and nursing staff about how your labor will be conducted. As you can imagine this isn't always straightforward, but the book will help you to pick your way through various possibilities.

Approaching motherhood

IN WRITING THIS BOOK, I have also taken into account the fact that for many women today motherhood comes rather later in life than it used to. It's now commonplace for a woman to pursue her career into her thirties and decide to have her first child somewhere around 35. The old obstetric concept of being an "elderly primipara" after the age of 30 is now outdated. With improvements to overall maternal health, doctors and midwives are used to dealing with first-time mothers in their late thirties and even early forties as a matter of routine, and see these pregnancies as normal rather than a cause for alarm.

Most women work for most of their pregnancy. This means that planning for a modern pregnancy and birth is quite different from that in the past when many women left work and stayed at home until they became pregnant. Now most women feel they have to give careful consideration to their future job security, and I have outlined the advantages and disadvantages in this book of combining work, pregnancy and motherhood. Even if you have organized to resume your job after, say, six months, you may find it impossible to leave your baby and decide to wait for a few months longer. No one knows before the birth of their own child just how they will feel in the event.

Every woman is beset by doubts, fears and anxieties—you would not be normal if you did not have them. Yet it will all seem easy and straightforward in retrospect. In the meantime, it's reassuring to think about the women all around you, hardly different from yourself, who are enjoying pregnancies, having memorable labors and births and, despite some sleepless nights, worries about feeds and weight gain, and who are thrilled with their babies. You, like them, will find that pregnancy and birth introduce you to a fulfilling phase of your life.

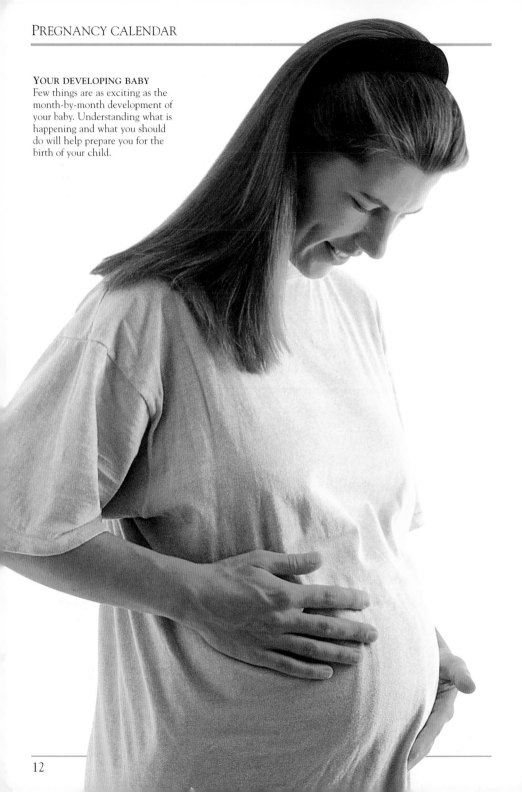

YOUR DEVELOPING BABY
Few things are as exciting as the month-by-month development of your baby. Understanding what is happening and what you should do will help prepare you for the birth of your child.

Pregnancy calendar

Knowing about the changes that happen during pregnancy helps you to become more aware of your body and your needs. It also helps you to remain calm if you understand that these changes, which aren't inevitable in all women, are perfectly normal. This month-by-month calendar summarizes the development of the baby and the changes in your body. However, every pregnancy is different; no two pregnancies develop at the same rate or feel the same, so don't be alarmed if you haven't experienced or noticed certain changes by the date given here.

Each month there is usually something else you need to be thinking about, such as booking your prenatal classes, starting to do special exercises, and buying maternity clothes and nursing bras. These are pointed out at the relevant time in the pregnancy calendar but are covered in greater detail in later chapters.

Becoming pregnant

SIGNS OF PREGNANCY

If you are planning a pregnancy and miss your period, you may suspect that you are pregnant. You may not notice any other changes apart from the missed period at first, but an increase in hormonal activity will confirm your pregnancy with one or more of the following physical signs:
● feeling of nausea at any time
● change in taste: perhaps you will suddenly not be able to tolerate alcohol or coffee
● a preference for certain foods, sometimes close to a craving
● a metallic taste in your mouth
● changes in your breasts; they may feel tender and tingly
● a need to urinate more frequently
● tiredness at any time of the day; you may even feel faint or dizzy too
● increase in normal vaginal discharge
● your emotions swing unpredictably.

DURATION OF PREGNANCY

Pregnancy lasts 266 days from the moment the egg is fertilized. However, actual fertilization is usually difficult to pinpoint precisely. When estimating how pregnant you are, day one of your pregnancy is taken from the first day of your last menstrual period (LMP) and not the day of fertilization. If you have an average 28-day cycle, fertilization is counted as having taken place around day 14 and not day one of your pregnancy. This is because ovulation usually takes place about 14 days before the start of your period.

The pregnancy timescale is thus 266 days plus 14 days—that is, 40 weeks. However, this is only a guide. The average normal pregnancy can last anything from 38 to 42 weeks. You can calculate your estimated date of delivery (EDD) by looking at the table on p. 49.

Weeks 6–10

By this time the uterus, which is usually the size and shape of a small pear, has become swollen and slightly enlarged, although it cannot yet be felt above the pubic bone. Increased blood flow to the cervix gives it the classic purplish tinge of pregnancy and it also becomes softened. Visit your doctor to confirm the pregnancy and have a preliminary discussion about the type of birth you wish to have (Chapter 3) and to arrange what sort of prenatal care you will receive, and where and how to book in (Chapter 4).

CONFIRMING YOUR PREGNANCY

- The pregnancy hormone human chorionic gonadotrophin (HCG) can be detected in tiny amounts in urine. Home kits, available from pharmacies, are 95 percent accurate and can confirm a pregnancy within a few days of your missed period. Another option is to go to your doctor's or a family planning clinic for a test.
- A blood test could reveal the pregnancy hormones within a few days of your missing a period.

DIAGNOSTIC TESTS

If you are 35 or over, your doctor will discuss with you the possibility of special tests—such as blood tests, ultrasound scans, CVS or amniocentesis (see pp. 78–81)—for any fetal disorders that can occur in older pregnant women or if there is a history of abnormality in your family.

PRENATAL CARE
The midwife will take your details when you book in (weeks 8–10).

TAKE CARE

The baby is most vulnerable in these first weeks, so you need to take precautions:
- Discuss any regular medication you may be taking before you try to conceive or as soon as you suspect you may be pregnant.
- Stop smoking and drinking alcohol.
- Find out if your work conditions are hazardous to your baby (see p. 45).
- If possible, check for rubella (German measles) immunity before you conceive (see p. 36).
- Keep high standards of hygiene with pets to avoid toxoplasmosis infection.

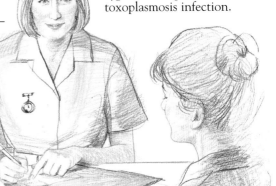

CHANGES TO YOUR BODY

Your breasts may be feeling tender and heavier and you may experience nausea in the morning or at any time of the day. Your emotions may be unpredictable because of hormone fluctuations and you may feel very tired, which can make your other symptoms feel more severe.

BABY'S DEVELOPMENT

The embryo, which can now be called a fetus, meaning "young one," has all the developing internal organs in place and is about the size of a small strawberry. The fetus is moving around a lot, though you cannot feel these movements yet.

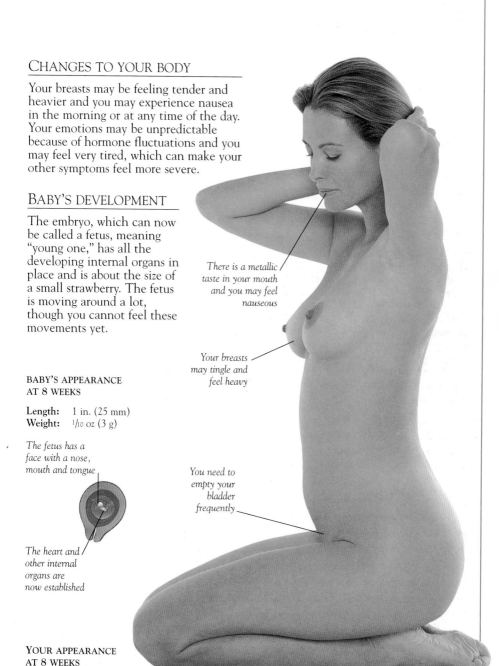

There is a metallic taste in your mouth and you may feel nauseous

Your breasts may tingle and feel heavy

You need to empty your bladder frequently

BABY'S APPEARANCE AT 8 WEEKS

Length: 1 in. (25 mm)
Weight: ¹/₁₀ oz (3 g)

The fetus has a face with a nose, mouth and tongue

The heart and other internal organs are now established

YOUR APPEARANCE AT 8 WEEKS

Week 12

After about 12 weeks of pregnancy, the irritation of complaints such as morning sickness and frequency of urination should have eased. You may notice a gain in weight for the first time. The amount of blood in your body increases steadily from now on so your heart and lungs have to work harder. Kidneys increase their work too. You may experience some constipation as the bowel slows down. Keep up your normal fitness routine after first checking with your doctor.

PRENATAL CARE

- You will attend your first prenatal clinic if you haven't already (see p. 74).
- You may be given an ultrasound scan to check for fetal abnormalities, if your baby is thought to be at risk (see p. 78).
- This is a good time to decide on your course of parenting classes. Classes organized by your hospital maternity unit are sometimes free. As well as providing information about pregnancy and birth, they help you to become familiar with hospital routines and the layout of the labor wards. You'll also have a chance to meet other parents whose babies are due at about the same time as yours.
- The midwife or healthcare professional can tell you about classes held locally either through the health center or privately (see p. 244 for addresses). Privately run classes are usually smaller and less formal, often taking place in the tutor's own home. They often specialize in prenatal exercises and techniques for managing labor with relaxation and breathing techniques (see p. 144).

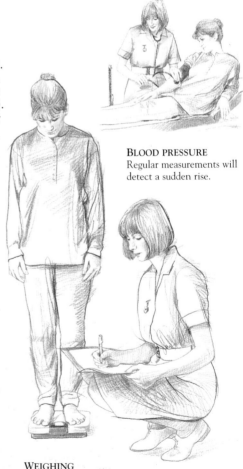

BLOOD PRESSURE
Regular measurements will detect a sudden rise.

WEIGHING
This happens when you visit.

CHANGES TO YOUR BODY

You should be feeling better as any nausea starts to diminish and you do not have to urinate so frequently. Constipation, however, may start to become a problem.

BABY'S DEVELOPMENT

The genital organs can now be seen clearly with ultrasound. The eyes are completely formed and the fingers and toes are developing, though they are still joined by webs of skin. Most of the internal organs are now working. The baby's movements are becoming stronger because his muscles are developing.

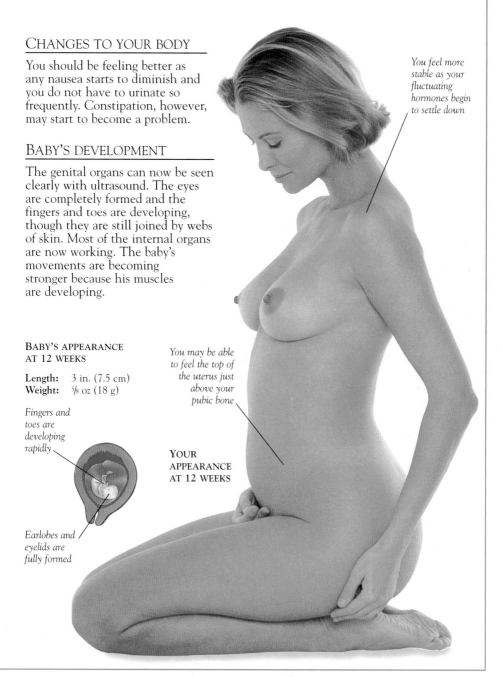

You feel more stable as your fluctuating hormones begin to settle down

BABY'S APPEARANCE AT 12 WEEKS

Length: 3 in. (7.5 cm)
Weight: ⅝ oz (18 g)

Fingers and toes are developing rapidly

Earlobes and eyelids are fully formed

You may be able to feel the top of the uterus just above your pubic bone

YOUR APPEARANCE AT 12 WEEKS

Week 16

You will start to feel better and more energetic. You will probably be noticeably pregnant now. Your muscles and ligaments begin to slacken and your waistline disappears. Choose your food carefully; your appetite will increase as you feel better and weight gain can be rapid. Start wearing comfortable, unrestricting clothes (see p. 136). If you haven't done so already, go out and buy a good bra with adequate support (see p. 137).

MEDICAL TESTS

● A screening blood test checks the level of alpha-fetoprotein (AFP) in your blood. If there is a higher or lower level than usual, this may indicate Down's syndrome or spina bifida in your baby so you may be scanned again or offered an amniocentesis at about 18 weeks. The results of the amniocentesis take about three weeks to come through (see p. 80).
● If you have had problems with an incompetent cervix before (see p. 158), a suture will be inserted at this stage under a general anesthetic.

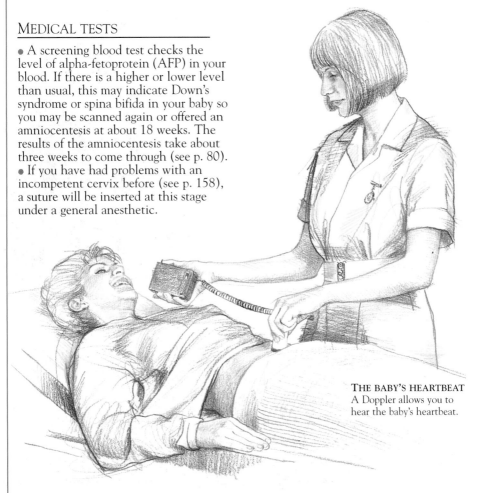

THE BABY'S HEARTBEAT
A Doppler allows you to hear the baby's heartbeat.

CHANGES TO YOUR BODY

You should be feeling much better than in the early stages of pregnancy and you will probably have more energy. You may notice changes in skin pigmentation on your face, breasts and arms.

BABY'S DEVELOPMENT

The baby is now fully formed—she even has distinctive fingerprints. As the tiny bones inside her ears harden, the baby can hear sounds, for example her mother's voice. Her movements become more vigorous and fine hair, known as lanugo, appears all over her body.

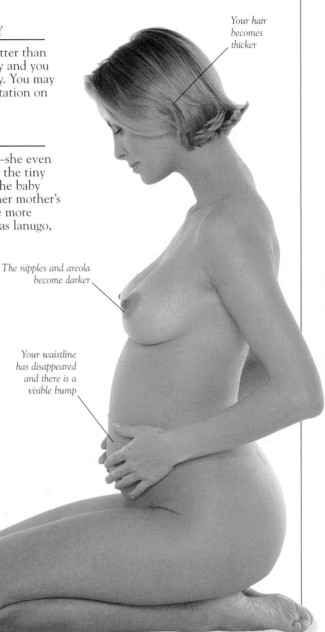

Your hair becomes thicker

The nipples and areola become darker

Your waistline has disappeared and there is a visible bump

BABY'S APPEARANCE AT 16 WEEKS

Length: 6 in. (16 cm)
Weight: 4 ¾ oz (135g)

The skin is transparent

Tiny fingernails are visible

The head appears large for the body

YOUR APPEARANCE AT 16 WEEKS

Week 20

By now you can feel your baby's movements as light, butterflylike ripples. You'll probably have an ultrasound scan at weeks 20–22, to check that the baby is growing normally. It will also show if there is more than one baby. If all is well you can enjoy the best part of your pregnancy. You should look radiant even though an increase in skin pigmentation may be more noticeable (see p. 100).

MIXED FEELINGS

It is normal for you and your partner to have mixed feelings about becoming parents. As you get nearer the birth your anxieties may increase as you question whether you are ready for parenthood and if it will change your lifestyle and your relationships. The best course of action is to talk these worries over. Another perspective is always valuable and may help you develop strategies.

TALK FRANKLY
Discuss your worries with your partner.

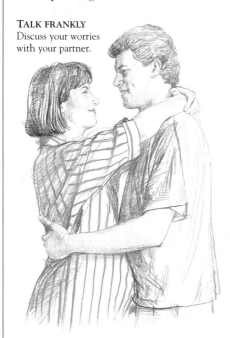

EXERCISES

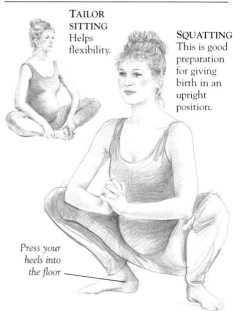

TAILOR SITTING
Helps flexibility.

SQUATTING
This is good preparation for giving birth in an upright position.

Press your heels into the floor

Exercise builds strong muscles to prepare you for labor so you should plan an exercise program at this time. At prenatal classes, which continue throughout pregnancy, you will be taught a number of exercises. You will learn how to clench your pelvic floor muscles (see p. 124) and increase your strength and flexibility in preparation for labor. You can also exercise by yourself. Swimming is excellent for general fitness and you are supported in the water as you do some of your prenatal exercises (see Chapter 9).

CHANGES TO YOUR BODY

You start to notice your baby's movements, which are felt as light flutters. Your breasts may produce colostrum, the first milk, and your gums may bleed. You may also experience nasal congestion. Some women have heavy vaginal discharge; if so, use a sanitary pad, not a tampon.

BABY'S DEVELOPMENT

The baby's teeth are forming in the jawbone, and, as his muscles develop, he is beginning to move about more vigorously in the womb. He will move in response to any pressure on the mother's abdomen.

**BABY'S APPEARANCE
AT 20 WEEKS**

Length: 10 in. (25 cm)
Weight: 12 oz (340 g)

*Skin may
darken in
patches*

*Breasts have
increased in size*

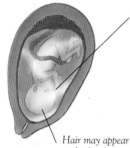

*The baby's
hands can
form fists*

*Stretchmarks
may appear on
your abdomen*

*Hair may appear
on his head*

**YOUR
APPEARANCE
AT 20 WEEKS**

Week 24

Your most rapid weight gain takes place around now; your feet will start to feel the strain and you should be conscious of your posture (see p. 120). Ensure that your shoes are comfortable and rest with your feet up when possible. By now your heart and lungs are doing 50 percent more work. Your increased fluid levels may cause you to feel hot and sweat more. Your face will look flushed because of increased blood circulation. If your baby was born now, she would be considered legally viable and could survive with care in a neonatal intensive care unit.

WEIGHT GAIN

You need to gain weight during pregnancy. Gone are the days when weight was watched obsessively and expectant mothers were admonished if they gained too much. Between weeks 24 and 32 there is usually the most rapid weight gain of pregnancy, but if you are already feeling heavy, this is the time to show some restraint or to increase your walking or swimming to use up any excess calories that you might have. However, now is not the time to try to diet. Eat a balanced variety of nutritious and fresh foods instead.

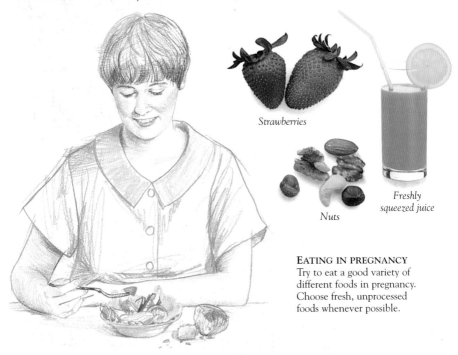

Strawberries

Nuts

Freshly squeezed juice

EATING IN PREGNANCY
Try to eat a good variety of different foods in pregnancy. Choose fresh, unprocessed foods whenever possible.

CHANGES TO YOUR BODY

By now you are visibly pregnant and need to wear loose-fitting clothes. You may feel hot and sweaty because of your increased blood supply. Some women experience rib pain because the baby is pressing upwards against the ribcage.

BABY'S DEVELOPMENT

Creases start to appear on the baby's palms and fingertips and she can suck her thumb. She can also hiccup. The baby's patterns of sleeping and activity seem random, but unfortunately she may be most active when you're trying to sleep. The nostrils open and she is making breathing motions.

Your face may look puffy because of water retention

Increased circulation may cause you to sweat more

BABY'S APPEARANCE AT 24 WEEKS

Length: 13 in. (33 cm)
Weight: 1 ¼ lb (570 g)

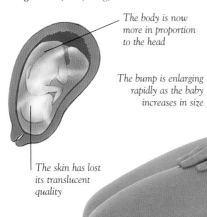

The body is now more in proportion to the head

The bump is enlarging rapidly as the baby increases in size

The skin has lost its translucent quality

YOUR APPEARANCE AT 24 WEEKS

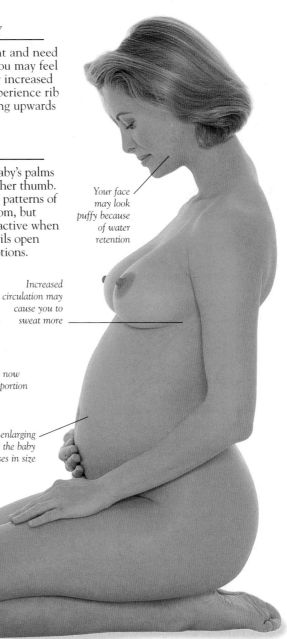

Week 28

You should tell your employer in writing when you plan to stop working (give three weeks' notice); when the baby is due; and when you plan to return to work. If born now, your baby has a more than 50 percent chance of survival if cared for in an appropriate unit.

PREGNANCY COMPLAINTS

Approach any minor discomforts of pregnancy sensibly (see Chapter 12) and be assured they will disappear after the birth. If indigestion troubles you, eat little and often and avoid problem foods. If you suffer from cramps, keep up your calcium intake with dairy products. Now is the time when the painless Braxton Hicks contractions start to become noticeable (see p. 97).

You should be getting plenty of rest and sleep. This is not always easy as your size, the baby's movements and any digestion problems make a continuous night's sleep almost impossible. Comfort in bed may help the problem; use pillows to wedge yourself into comfortable positions for sleep at night and during your rest in the day.

COMFORTABLE POSITION
This is a good position to rest in during the day.

CLOTHING

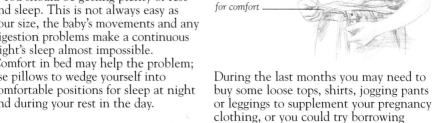

YOUR WARDROBE
Many of your normal casual clothes can be worn in pregnancy.

Choose drawstring waistbands for comfort

During the last months you may need to buy some loose tops, shirts, jogging pants or leggings to supplement your pregnancy clothing, or you could try borrowing clothes from your partner. For special occasions you may want to buy some maternity wear. Maternity dresses are usually longer in the front to allow for the bump. Wear sensible footwear such as low-heeled, comfortable shoes.

CHANGES TO YOUR BODY

As you become bigger, you may notice stretchmarks on your stomach or thighs and some women experience lower back pain which is caused by the enlarging abdomen and loosening of the pelvic joints. As the uterus expands, you may have some heartburn or indigestion.

BABY'S DEVELOPMENT

Fat is building up under the baby's skin and he is coated in a waxy substance called vernix, which protects the skin so that it doesn't get soggy in the amniotic fluid. His eyes are open and he can see.

The veins on your breasts become noticeable

BABY'S APPEARANCE AT 28 WEEKS

The womb has risen halfway between your navel and breastbone

Length: 14 ½ in. (37 cm)
Weight: 2 lb (900 g)

He has less room to move and wriggles if you are in a position that he doesn't like

His lungs are now fully developed

YOUR APPEARANCE AT 28 WEEKS

Week 32

If you exert yourself too much you will feel exhausted and breathless. You are probably looking forward to stopping work and should try to rest during the day if possible. Take things easy, especially if you aren't sleeping well. Parenting classes will begin soon and you can prepare yourself by gathering all the necessary items for the birth (see p. 168) and by going shopping for the baby too. You may have another blood test at your prenatal clinic to check that you aren't anemic (see p. 156) and that there aren't any Rhesus problems (see p. 162).

GOOD POSTURE

Stresses and strains are put on all your joints and ligaments during pregnancy. The change in your center of gravity as the uterus enlarges can affect your posture, and if you don't concentrate and think about your body when you pick things up and carry heavy bags, for example, you could suffer from unnecessary back pain.

TIREDNESS

Difficulty in sleeping is very common at this stage of pregnancy. If you find yourself lying awake, use this time to practice your relaxation techniques. Hot water bottles help soothe ribcage or pelvic pain. If you wake because you need to urinate, rock gently backwards and forwards while emptying your bladder. This will help to empty it more thoroughly, and should increase the interval before you need to get up again.

SEX DURING PREGNANCY

Sex in late pregnancy becomes difficult because of your size so you may need to find more comfortable positions (see p. 107) or find other ways of loving. Massage not only soothes aches and pains but can be a positive way of showing affection.

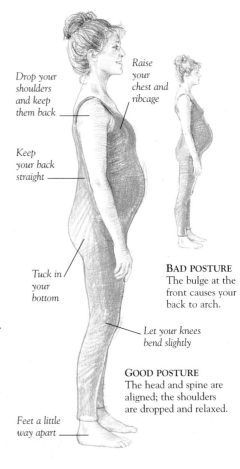

Drop your shoulders and keep them back

Raise your chest and ribcage

Keep your back straight

Tuck in your bottom

Feet a little way apart

BAD POSTURE
The bulge at the front causes your back to arch.

Let your knees bend slightly

GOOD POSTURE
The head and spine are aligned; the shoulders are dropped and relaxed.

CHANGES TO YOUR BODY

Your lower ribcage may feel sore and you
may need to urinate more often as the
uterus expands, putting pressure on your
internal organs and diaphragm. Your navel
will look flattened and the linea nigra may
be visible running down your abdomen.

BABY'S DEVELOPMENT

Most babies will have turned head downwards (cephalic position) in preparation for
birth. If she was born now, the baby would
have at least an 80 percent chance of
survival because her lungs have developed.
The placenta has now reached maturity.

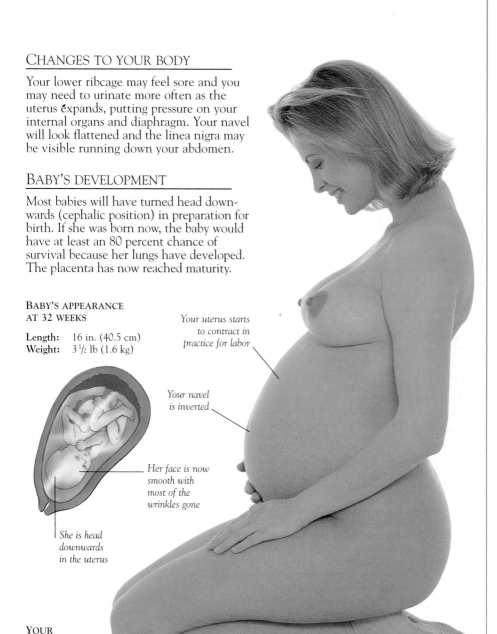

**BABY'S APPEARANCE
AT 32 WEEKS**

Length: 16 in. (40.5 cm)
Weight: 3 ½ lb (1.6 kg)

*Your uterus starts
to contract in
practice for labor*

*Your navel
is inverted*

*Her face is now
smooth with
most of the
wrinkles gone*

*She is head
downwards
in the uterus*

**YOUR
APPEARANCE
AT 32 WEEKS**

Week 36

By now you should be planning your life carefully; don't organize too much activity, instead keep yourself entertained with gentle pastimes. Get others to do all the running around. Strong Braxton Hicks contractions may make you believe you are in labor (see p. 173). Practice your breathing techniques with the Braxton Hicks.

Prenatal clinics will be at least every two weeks until delivery. If this is your first baby, the head will "engage"—drop into the pelvic cavity; this eases breathing problems but pain may be felt in the pelvic region. Avoid standing as your ankles might swell. If you have a heavy vaginal discharge, wear light stick-on sanitary pads (never internal tampons).

BREASTFEEDING BRAS

Your breasts won't enlarge any more until the milk comes in shortly after the birth. If you plan to breastfeed, now is the time to buy at least two front-opening nursing bras.

Wearing an ordinary pregnancy bra, measure yourself with a tape measure, noting both the size and cup sizes. If you like, you can ask the shop assistant to measure you, or if you are not sure which sort of bra you prefer, you can ask for advice. If colostrum is secreted, you may need to wear breast pads to prevent stains on your clothing.

PREPARATION FOR BIRTH

The nesting instinct becomes strong in the last trimester. You will probably have the time now that you have stopped work to buy clothes for the baby and prepare a room with a crib, changing pad, diapers and other necessary items (see Chapter 14). This nesting instinct can lead to bursts of activity but try not to overdo it. You will need all your strength later for labor and birth. Around this time you also need to prepare clothes and other items you will need for your delivery (see pp. 168–169).

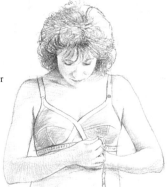

BRA SIZE
To find your bra size, measure under your breasts.

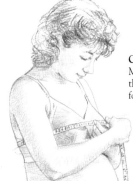

CUP SIZE
Measure around the fullest part for cup size.

CHANGES TO YOUR BODY

As the baby's head drops into your pelvic cavity, irritating digestive problems and feelings of breathlessness should lessen. It may be more difficult for you to get a good night's sleep as your large abdomen makes it difficult to find a comfortable position.

BABY'S DEVELOPMENT

The baby is steadily putting on weight. He may now have lots of hair and his fingernails have grown to reach the end of his fingers. The irises of his eyes are blue.

You may have backache and stiff joints

BABY'S APPEARANCE AT 36 WEEKS

Length: 18 in. (46 cm)
Weight: 5 ½ lb (2.5 kg)

His body is plump and round

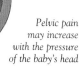

Pelvic pain may increase with the pressure of the baby's head

He has shed most of the fine hair (lanugo)

YOUR
APPEARANCE
AT 36 WEEKS

Week 40

The expected date of delivery is near and you may become anxious when it passes. Don't worry, however, as only five percent of babies arrive on the due date. You will be feeling very heavy and tired; all your movements will be an effort, and as the baby is lying deep in your pelvis, you may have pain in the groin and pins and needles down your legs. The baby's movements decrease in force (although not in frequency) because there is less space for her in the uterus. Most babies lie head down ready for birth.

SIGNS OF LABOR

The Braxton Hicks contractions may be so strong that you think you are in labor. If in doubt, call the hospital or speak to your midwife. True contractions are more regular than Braxton Hicks. Labor isn't always signaled by a definite sign (see p. 173). You may have a "show" of blood-tinged gelatinous mucus that has blocked the cervix during pregnancy. This show may occur up to two weeks before the onset of true labor, but is a sign that it is not far off. Other signs are:
- a leakage of amniotic fluid; it may be a gush or just a trickle
- contractions occurring at regular intervals.

TIMING CONTRACTIONS

Severe Braxton Hicks contractions can often be mistaken for labor. However, if you time the contractions over an hour, noting when each one starts and how long it lasts, you can find out whether this is true labor. The contractions should become stronger, more frequent (see below) and last for between 30 and 60 seconds. Sometimes contractions start and then fade away. You should plan to go to the hospital when they are about five minutes apart.

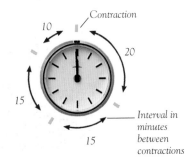

Contraction

10

20

15

15

Interval in minutes between contractions

CHANGES TO YOUR BODY

You are feeling very tired and all your movements take a lot of extra effort. Your lower abdomen feels very heavy and your skin is tight and uncomfortable. You may want to clean the house in readiness for the birth, but try to conserve your energy.

BABY'S DEVELOPMENT

The baby is full size and, if it is a boy, the testicles will usually have descended. If this is your first baby, the head will have already engaged in the pelvis.

BABY'S APPEARANCE AT 40 WEEKS

Length: 20 in. (51 cm)
Weight: 7½ lb (3.4 kg)

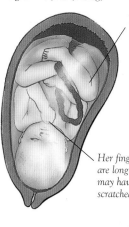

Your skin feels tight and itchy

Most of the vernix has gone, but some may still be present in skin folds

Your cervix is softening in preparation for labor

Her fingernails are long and she may have scratched herself

You may have pins and needles

YOUR APPEARANCE AT 40 WEEKS

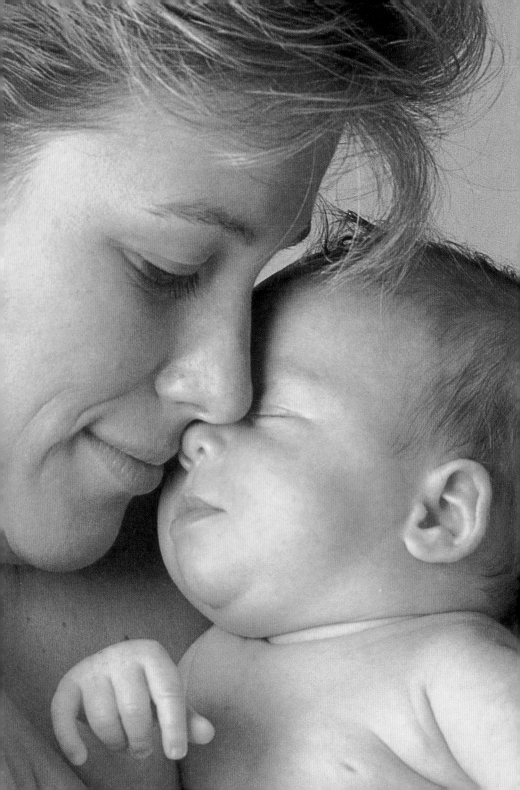

Becoming a mother

I mmediately after the birth you will probably be tired, but many women feel elated and full of energy. Everyone reacts differently. You'll certainly be lighter and less ungainly. If you're in a hospital there will be the ward routines to deal with, but once you're home, you can enjoy the peace and security of familiar surroundings and get to know your baby. Life for the next few weeks will revolve around the baby, but in time both of you, together with your partner and any other children in your family, should begin to adjust to a more settled routine (Chapter 17).

YOUR NEW BABY

At birth, your baby may have lots of hair, or be quite bald. He may not look quite as you expected, but as the days go by any marks or bruising from the birth will fade. The content of your baby's first bowel movement after birth is called meconium, a dark, greenish, sticky substance. This will change gradually to more normal bowel movements once feeding starts.

Immediately after birth, the baby will be tested and given an Apgar score (see p. 218). This gives an indication of his general well-being. Later on he will be weighed and measured, and your midwife will continue to do this regularly for the first ten days or so. The doctor will give your baby a general examination to check for any abnormality.

Around the sixth day after the birth, a blood sample is taken from your baby's heel. This checks for PKU (phenylketonuria) and congenital hypothyroidism, both of which are rare causes of mental disability that can be treated if detected.

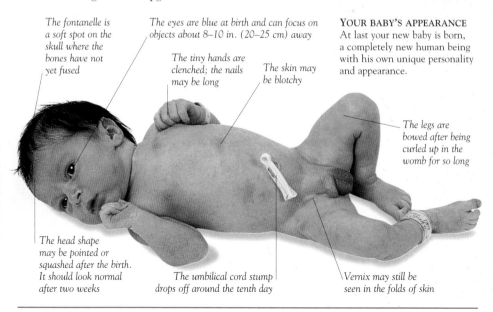

The fontanelle is a soft spot on the skull where the bones have not yet fused

The eyes are blue at birth and can focus on objects about 8–10 in. (20–25 cm) away

The tiny hands are clenched; the nails may be long

The skin may be blotchy

YOUR BABY'S APPEARANCE
At last your new baby is born, a completely new human being with his own unique personality and appearance.

The legs are bowed after being curled up in the womb for so long

The head shape may be pointed or squashed after the birth. It should look normal after two weeks

The umbilical cord stump drops off around the tenth day

Vernix may still be seen in the folds of skin

1

Deciding to have a baby

The professor of obstetrics at my medical school used to tell us that there was no right time to have a baby because something else always came up in a couple's professional or domestic life. The corollary of this is that there is no wrong time to have a baby either. Paramount in the decision to have a baby, however, is that it is wanted; ideally it should also be planned. Even planning is often not as perfect as we would like nor, in my opinion, should it be. For one thing couples may not find it easy to conceive once they have made the decision.

When I decided to have my first child, I stopped taking the oral contraceptive pill and was pregnant the next month. When I wanted my second child, however, I failed to conceive for 12 months and they were 12 months of anguish. So be prepared for the best planning to go awry.

Are you healthy enough?

EVERY YEAR A SMALL NUMBER of babies are born who are not as healthy as they might be. There are many reasons why this may happen, but two of the most important factors are the nutrition and fitness of the mother. Although it has been shown that maternal malnutrition and lack of fitness become more common as you descend the economic scale, it is also worth bearing in mind that eating disorders or excessive dieting may also have an effect on your health. Try to pay attention to nutrition and lifestyle as well as your general state of health *before* you decide to have a baby (see p. 113).

DIET

If you're not already doing so, you can improve your health enormously by examining your diet. You may think you eat well but look closely. Do you skip breakfast and eat a small lunch, saving your appetite for an evening meal? Do you leave the fresh fruit for your children? Do you resort to high-calorie snacks to get you through the day? You can improve your health almost immediately by increasing your intake of fresh fruit, vegetables and high-fiber foods and cutting out highly refined, starchy foods (see pp. 108–113).

FOLIC ACID

It's now known that sufficient folic acid is important in reducing the risk of spinal abnormalities in the fetus. Take folic acid supplements for at least three months before you start trying for a baby (400 mcg per day is the recommended dose), and eat plenty of foods rich in folic acid such as dark-green leafy vegetables, bread, cereals and some nuts (but avoid peanuts). If your baby was unplanned, start taking folic acid as soon as you know you're pregnant. Continue to take folic acid throughout your pregnancy.

EXERCISE

If you lead a sedentary life you should try to fit in some kind of exercise, either a sport such as tennis, swimming or jogging, or an exercise program using a rowing

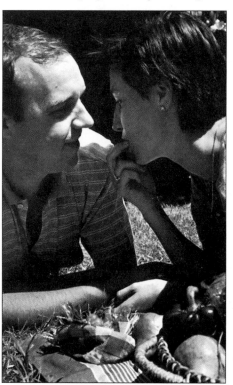

machine or an exercise bicycle. Try to take some form of exercise for a minimum of 20 minutes a time at least four times a week, during which you should get slightly out of breath and sweat a bit. If this sounds daunting, start with a brisk walk, which is better than nothing.

SMOKING, ALCOHOL AND DRUGS

You should take particular care to cut down on "social" drugs before you conceive, especially cigarettes (see p. 117). Smoking is associated with infertility in women, though the effects on male fertility may be more damaging. Sperm are more at risk than eggs from the chemicals in cigarette smoke and it is believed that smoking could cause damage to chromosomes in the cells of smokers.

The risks of smoking to the unborn baby are well documented. It is now known that passive smoking can be as harmful as smoking itself; a woman living or working with people who smoke inhales a lot of nicotine and tars from the cigarette smoke in the air around her.

There is research that suggests that alcohol is also riskier at the time of conception and during the early weeks than was previously thought. Alcohol is increasingly being linked to certain birth defects and in severe cases to a syndrome producing physical and mental abnormalities (see p. 118). To be on the safe side, avoid drinking alcohol if you are trying for a baby.

It is also risky to take recreational drugs in pregnancy. Cannabis is known to interfere with the normal production of male sperm and increases the risk of conceiving a baby with chromosomal abnormalities. It is also thought that LSD can cause birth defects if it is taken around the time of conception.

HEALTHY LIVING
Eating a good balanced diet, taking plenty of exercise and fresh air and finding the time to relax when you're away from work will improve your chances of conceiving a healthy baby.

AGE OF THE PARENTS

Age will always be a factor for you to consider when deciding to have a baby but not the negative one that you might think. Considerations of personal freedom and career moves are causing more and more women to wait until they are over 30 to become pregnant but many still fear that they may be leaving it too late. This is because they may have heard that the longer they wait the greater is the chance of having a difficult pregnancy or even, possibly, a child with an abnormality. However, although the risk of having a Down's syndrome baby, for example, increases with the age of the mother (see p. 81), carefully documented case studies show that it is not physically dangerous to the woman herself if she defers pregnancy until she is past her twenties.

The risks undoubtedly do increase with age but every decision to have a child is unique and the age of the parents is only one factor, and a very small one, in weighing up the risks and benefits. The age of the father relates more to infertility than to a risk factor. Many other factors affect the risk factor ratio in each woman's case. Of course, what these statistics do is to lump all mothers over the age of, say, 30 together, regardless of their health or financial background, whereas an important factor in maternal risk is the mother's socioeconomic situation. The complications during pregnancy and delivery for this group are not related to age but to other factors such as malnutrition; an individual pregnant woman will only need special care if she is poorly nourished, regardless of her age (see p. 34).

Many experts have come up with the "best" age to have a baby but in most cases, however, women don't take this into consideration. Although physically a woman may be better suited to childbirth in her early twenties, emotionally she may not be ready to be a parent. When she is younger a woman may be too involved with her career to have children or she may not have met the right person to be the father of her children. Many women simply are not ready to settle down until they are over 30.

Though fertility does diminish with age (see p. 44), an important factor to consider is that the statistics show that the odds are greatly in favor of your having a successful pregnancy at almost any age provided you are healthy. Many studies have been done on normal pregnancies in women past the age of 50 and all of them concluded that the general health of the mother is much more important than age alone as a factor in predicting how the pregnancy will turn out—so remember if your health is good, the decision to have a baby should not be abandoned on account of age alone.

RUBELLA

If your developing baby is exposed to the German measles (rubella) virus, malformations, including deafness, blindness and heart disease, may occur. This is particularly likely during the first three months, when all the vital organs are forming and developing.

What to do

If you did not have German measles as a child and were not vaccinated against it at puberty, consult your doctor before you try for a baby and ask for a blood test to find out if you're immune. If you aren't immune, ask to be vaccinated against rubella, and then wait at least three months before trying to conceive. If you're already pregnant, a blood test will show if you have some immunity. However, even if vaccinated you may not be completely immune so if you come into contact with the disease, tell your doctor at once, though unfortunately contact is most hazardous before the rash appears. If you are infected, you may want to discuss the difficult decision about whether to terminate your pregnancy.

PREEXISTING MEDICAL CONDITIONS

Some women's general medical condition—including diabetes, heart disease and Rhesus incompatibility (see pp. 156–163)—may make the pregnancy and labor difficult. If you have any of these conditions, you should be able to have a normal birth with careful prenatal care and monitoring, and perhaps observation in the hospital prenatal ward during the last trimester of your pregnancy. If you're undertaking a long-term drug treatment, for epilepsy as an example, talk to your doctor about your treatment before trying for a baby.

Effects on lifestyle

A SURVEY DONE in America showed that the number of women who considered motherhood the most pleasurable aspect of being a woman had dropped in the last 20 years, while the number of women who opted for work as being more fulfilling had risen. As women in the West have reexamined their status in society and decided to be more self-determined than they have been in the past, aided by reliable contraceptive methods, fewer are taking the role of wife and mother as the automatic choice in life. The investment of more time in the pursuit of a career also means that more women are opting to have families later in their lives.

For most women, having children is now a matter of choice and planning, and their decision to be a mother is a well-considered one, although unfortunately too many teenage girls still become pregnant by accident. Nowadays, few people would subscribe to the unquestioned idealization of the act of childbearing that once made society view it as essential to women's fulfillment.

Some women, as they get older and fear that their fertility is diminishing, regard single parenthood as a possible choice even though they may not have found a partner with whom they wish to settle down. Women who make this decision and conceive a baby are usually remarkable for their single-mindedness and are quite prepared to face the implications of being a lone mother. To them motherhood is a chosen state, not one imposed by chance.

ANXIETY ABOUT PARENTHOOD

When you consider the change in lifestyle, the possible disruption of a happy relationship, the concessions and adjustments that have to be made with the advent of a baby, the decision not to have children at all becomes more understandable than it might have been. Many people fear parenthood and it's a reasonable anxiety. It's natural to worry about coping with your child's upbringing and what you will do if things go wrong.

There may be economic pressures, the problem of resuming your career and possible frustration due to loss of freedom. Not everyone relishes the fact that they are no longer free agents and you'd be quite normal if you questioned your ability to feel loving and caring towards your baby all the time. In normal life you are besieged by many negative feelings such as resentment, bad temper, or frustration, and there's no reason to think that the presence of your baby will call an end to these feelings.

It is perhaps only when you become a parent that you realize how much is demanded of you. In the early years your baby is an unscrupulous taker. But the one lesson that I have learned is that the more you give the more is given back to you as your child grows older.

FATHER'S ROLE

The role of the modern father has changed too. The majority of fathers take the responsibility of being a parent very seriously and they are not prepared to be strangers to their children. For many years men were shut out of pregnancy and from the day-to-day care of their children on the assumption that it was woman's work and that it was not their place. But now liberated mothers have fostered liberated fathers. These fathers feel free to indulge all their paternal instincts, and they want to be involved with their partners during pregnancy and delivery and are not prepared to miss out on their children's growing up. The modern father is an active father rather than a passive one.

Even in the early years your child will reward you with irreplaceable moments of pleasure, possibly pride, and as she grows older, with more and more hours of companionship, love, comfort and joy. Most fathers who have a keen interest in the pregnancy stay interested after the baby is born. Studies have shown that a father becomes more closely attached to his baby according to how much he holds it during the first six weeks of life and whether he answers the baby's cry. His attitude is also affected by his partner's enjoyment of pregnancy and motherhood. The happier a man is about his partner's pregnancy, the more he shares in the monitoring of her prenatal care and the more he looks forward to enjoying fatherhood, the more he will get out of the first few weeks of his baby's life.

SHARING RESPONSIBILITIES

Many couples agree that parents should be equal and the roles of parenting and childrearing must be equally shared, if possible. When you decide to have a baby you and your partner should view it as a contract: a contract which states that you are equally responsible for rearing the child you have conceived.

Try to discuss and agree with each other about the roles that you are going to play. Most women no longer expect to be the sole nursemaid, childminder and baby-sitter, confined to the house with its limited horizons and interests while the father leaves home early to work and doesn't return until the baby is asleep. More and more women—and men—are unwilling to be partners in this kind of arrangement. These are some of the points that must be resolved between you before the baby is born if you want to provide a happy and stable environment in which to rear your child.

Stopping contraception

IF YOU ARE TAKING the oral contraceptive pill, you should plan to have three normal menstrual periods before you become pregnant to allow your metabolic functions to return to normal after coming off the pill. During the intervening months you will need to use some mechanical form of contraception such as condoms or a diaphragm (see p. 235).

Much has been written about a woman's return to fertility after taking the pill, particularly for long periods of time. Originally it was thought that fertility was increased after stopping the pill as the body overcompensated for long periods of suppressed fertility. We now know that this is not necessarily so, but the majority of women conceive in the first year after stopping the pill and nearly all women after two years.

If you suspect that you have become pregnant while taking the pill, consult your doctor at once as there's a slight risk to the embryo from the hormones in the oral contraceptive pill.

There's no need to put off conception after having an IUD (coil) removed. If you become pregnant with one in place, your doctor won't try to remove it as it may be difficult, and the risk of precipitating a miscarriage is greater than if it is left in place.

Becoming pregnant

KNOWING ABOUT your natural body cycles will give you enough information both to conceive and to avoid conception. The three body rhythms that you can observe are your monthly menstrual cycles, your daily body temperature and the appearance and consistency of the cervical mucus (your vaginal discharge).

OBSERVING BODY RHYTHMS

Women have menstrual cycles of varying length. After recording your menstrual cycles, say for four months, you may find that the shortest one was 26 days and the longest one was 32 days.

RECORD OF MENSTRUAL CYCLE

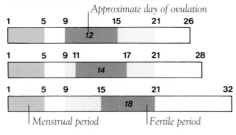

Approximate day of ovulation

Using the chart above you can see that your fertile days are from the 9th to the 21st day of each cycle, since ovulation normally occurs 14 days before menstruation. For conception, these are the days to concentrate on. A woman's body temperature drops and then rises just before ovulation. Take your temperature each morning before you get out of bed and chart it on a daily temperature chart (see below) for several months. A regular pattern will soon emerge. You are fertile for one day before the temperature drops and for one day after it remains elevated.

Your vaginal discharge (mucus) goes through a cycle of changes as the month progresses. Just after menstruation there is hardly any mucus but it is cloudy, sticky and thick. As you approach the fertile period it becomes abundant, clear and stretchy. As soon as you notice this change you've entered your fertile period. Fertility wanes when the mucus becomes cloudy, sticky and thick once again.

FREQUENCY OF INTERCOURSE

Conception is not helped by frequent intercourse. The more often a man ejaculates the fewer sperm are contained in his ejaculate and the number may drop below the minimum required for conception. If you're trying for a baby, it's a good idea for your partner to abstain from ejaculation for a few days before your fertile period to allow sperm numbers to rise and to have intercourse no more than once daily during your fertile days.

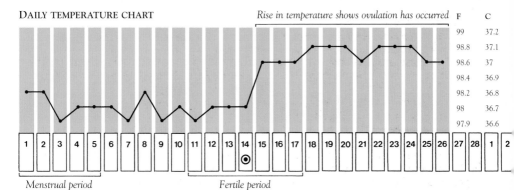

DAILY TEMPERATURE CHART

Rise in temperature shows ovulation has occurred

Menstrual period   Fertile period

INFLUENCE OF CHROMOSOMES AND GENES

Each cell in the body contains 46 chromosomes in 23 pairs, one half of each pair coming from the father's sperm and the other half from the mother's ovum. Each chromosome consists of two chains (known as the double helix) of thousands of genes strung together.

One pair of the 23 pairs of chromosomes determines gender. This pair is either XX (female) or XY (male), made up from donations from the mother and father. A mother only donates an X chromosome in her eggs, but a father can donate either X or Y, because a man produces two kinds of sperm—X (female) or Y (male). Biologically the male is responsible for the sex of the baby. If a Y sperm unites with the ovum, the baby will be a boy (XY), but if it's an X that unites with the ovum, the baby will be a girl (XX). Scientists have discovered that the Y sperm is produced in greater numbers, has a longer tail and moves faster than the X sperm, but the X sperm survives longer. Although there is no guarantee it will work,

if you want a boy, you could have sex as near as possible to the day you ovulate; and for a girl, a few days before ovulation.

A gene is a minute unit of DNA (deoxyribonucleic acid). Genes direct the development of all the body's organs and systems and determine the intellectual and physical characteristics we derive from our parents. Characteristics such as the color of the eyes and hair have a gene from the mother and father. Each characteristic has a dominant and recessive form. The gene for dark hair, for example, is always dominant over the gene for blond hair, and the gene for brown eyes will always dominate the one for blue. However, both genes are present, though one is masked. This is why two dark-haired parents can have a blond child in whom hair color is represented by the masked blond from the mother and the masked blond from the father.

GENETIC INHERITANCE
If both brown-haired parents are carrying the masked gene for fair hair, their children may be blond.

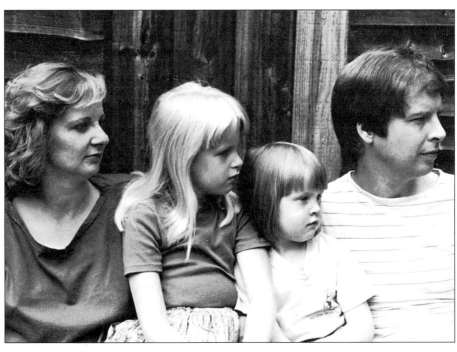

Genetic counseling

Quite rightly, emphasis is put on the mother's health because it is crucial to give the baby a healthy environment in which to develop. But the health of the father is crucial too. Only healthy men produce healthy sperm, with large numbers of normal sperm. This gives the best possible chance for a healthy union between the egg and one of the father's sperm. If either the sperm or the egg is defective, they may not be able to unite at all. If they are only slightly defective it is possible for a baby to develop that is not completely normal.

Some conditions are due to abnormalities of the chromosomes. Chromosome counts may give you some idea of the likelihood of conceiving a child who will suffer from the disease. This simple, painless procedure involves some cells being gently scraped from the inside of your mouth which are then examined under a microscope.

Every year thousands of children are born with congenital malformations, but the majority of these cannot be anticipated. If,

however, there is a history with either partner of a disease or condition that runs through family members and generations, then you should seek genetic counseling. Conditions that run in families include hemophilia, cystic fibrosis and muscular dystrophy. Having a baby is by no means ruled out if there is a hereditary tendency to a particular condition, but your decision to go ahead and try can only be helped by having a specialist investigation and counseling to determine the risk, depending on whether the affected gene is recessive (such as with cystic fibrosis) or dominant (Huntington's chorea).

Everyone takes some risk, albeit a minute one, when they decide to have a baby. Knowing how your risk compares to everyone else's is information that you cannot do without. If it's a small risk, you may decide to go ahead and try. If, however, the risk is very great, you may decide that you would prefer to try to adopt a child.

HIV/AIDS

It is important that you know how to protect yourself against the HIV virus that leads to AIDS, and to be assertive about it. All women should insist on safe sex and any new sexual encounter should be prefaced by a frank discussion about HIV/AIDS. Over three-quarters of women who become infected with the HIV virus acquire it heterosexually, there being no particular social pattern. The risk varies from person to person and partner to partner—some women do not become infected after hundreds of contacts, while others are infected after one.

When a virus gets into the body the blood makes a substance called an antibody. People who have been infected with HIV produce antibodies to the virus and, when tested, are said to be HIV positive. Because the mother's antibodies can cross the placenta, all babies born to HIV-positive mothers will also show up as HIV positive,

but not all of these babies will be infected. Some time between the ages of six and 18 months many babies will lose their mothers' antibodies and, once tested as HIV negative, they are then presumed to be uninfected.

More sensitive tests are now being used to allow a diagnosis of HIV infection to be made in the first few months of life. Even if the baby is found to be HIV positive, a good many babies survive into later childhood, although a third of HIV positive babies die before the age of two.

If you think you may be HIV positive, you can request a blood test to check. If you are found to be HIV positive, you should be counseled about the likelihood of contracting full-blown AIDS, and also about your own risk of transmitting the virus to the baby. There are now treatments available that reduce the risk of a mother infecting her baby.

Fertilization

IF YOUR MENSTRUAL CYCLE is regular, as a general rule fertilization happens about a week after you have finished menstruating or 14 days before your next period begins. About seven to 10 days after this, the fertilized ovum is implanted in the lining of the womb. By the end of another week it is firmly attached by its primitive placenta which links the developing embryo to its mother (see p. 83). The placenta is the organ through which foodstuffs and oxygen are carried from the mother to the baby and waste substances are carried from the baby to the mother. It is an absolutely crucial organ to the healthy progress of pregnancy because it produces pregnancy hormones that are responsible for maintaining the health of the developing baby, the uterus and the female genital organs. These hormones also prepare the woman's body for labor and for birth.

The ovum is usually fertilized about a third of the way along the fallopian tube by a single sperm which was deposited with millions of others in the vagina after ejaculation. Within a few seconds of ejaculation the sperm become mobile with the lashings of their whiplike tails. This then carries them at top speed out of the acid conditions of the vagina and through the neck of the cervix, which has become more fluid during ovulation, into the cavity of the uterus. In a few

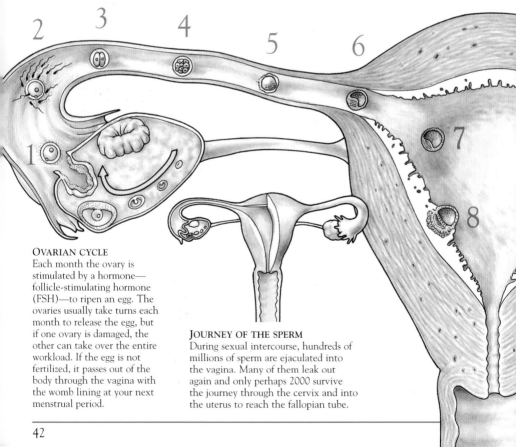

OVARIAN CYCLE
Each month the ovary is stimulated by a hormone—follicle-stimulating hormone (FSH)—to ripen an egg. The ovaries usually take turns each month to release the egg, but if one ovary is damaged, the other can take over the entire workload. If the egg is not fertilized, it passes out of the body through the vagina with the womb lining at your next menstrual period.

JOURNEY OF THE SPERM
During sexual intercourse, hundreds of millions of sperm are ejaculated into the vagina. Many of them leak out again and only perhaps 2000 survive the journey through the cervix and into the uterus to reach the fallopian tube.

seconds the sperm pass through the uterus and enter the fallopian tube to meet the ovum that is traveling down the tube towards them. Sperm are chemically attracted to the comparatively enormous ovum and attach themselves to it like limpets over the whole surface. However, only one sperm pierces the outer coat of the ovum. Instantly the egg loses its attraction, hardens its outer shell and all the superfluous sperm let go. This whole process, from ejaculation to fertilization, can take less than 60 minutes.

A ripe ovum usually survives for only 12 hours, and a maximum of 24. Sperm retain the power to fertilize for not much longer than 24 hours; 36 hours is probably about the limit. Fertilization is therefore unlikely unless sexual intercourse occurs one or two days before or immediately after ovulation.

Only the head of the sperm fuses with the ovum, forming a single cell. The cell divides into two in the first 24 hours; by the fourth day it is a ball of over 100 cells. This ball of cells floats free for the first three days in the cavity of the uterus, nurtured on uterine "milk" secreted by glands in the uterine wall. By the end of the first week, it has implanted into the uterine lining, where it is continuously bathed in a lake of its mother's blood, allowing food and waste to pass to and fro. Until week 8 the developing baby is known as an embryo, after which it is called a fetus, Latin for "young one."

1 The ovum is liberated from the surface of the ovary around the 14th day of the menstrual cycle. It is caught in the funnel-shaped end of the fallopian tube and is propeled along it by muscular contractions.

2 Fertilization by one sperm usually occurs about a third of the way along the tube.

3 The fertilized cell (known as a zygote) divides in two within 24 hours.

4 With repeated cell divisions a ball of cells is formed.

5 The egg continues to divide as it is swept along the tube.

6 A hollow cavity, filled with fluid, starts to form in the ball of cells. This is known as a blastocyst.

7 The blastocyst reaches the cavity of the uterus.

8 Implantation begins around day 7 and is most commonly in the upper part of the uterus on the side nearest the ovary. By day 10 the embryo has become firmly embedded.

CONCEPTION OF TWINS

When a single egg released from the ovary is fertilized, divides into two cells which then separate, this results in the development of identical twins; they are the same sex and usually share the same placenta. More commonly (in 70 percent of twins) two separate eggs may be fertilized by two different sperm. These are "fraternal twins" and usually have separate placentas and amniotic sacs.

IDENTICAL TWINS   FRATERNAL TWINS

Once the egg has been fertilized it splits into separate cells. This split may occur after implantation in the uterus.

Most twins occur when two eggs are released into the fallopian tube and are fertilized by two separate sperm.

Infertility

OVER SIX MILLION WOMEN in the United States are subfertile and unable to have babies. The ratio of one in ten is fairly constant throughout the Western nations. Infertility, however, is not a matter of either partner exclusively but of the couple as a unit. In some circumstances the high fertility of one partner can compensate for the low fertility of the other. On the other hand, marginal fertility in both partners may result in sterility. This would explain the paradox of a childless couple splitting up and then both partners producing children without any difficulty in a new partnership.

FEMALE INFERTILITY

In women one of the most important factors that affects fertility is age. Fertility begins to diminish around the age of 25. After the age of 45 only half a woman's cycles are ovulatory, so she has only half as many fertile periods during the year as a younger woman. The decline in a man's fertility is more gradual. It is the same as a woman's at the age of 20 and wanes slowly to 10 percent by the age of 60.

In many women the desire for children can be intense and overriding. Many women become physically ill with the desire to conceive. I well understand and sympathize with this uncontrollable desire. I myself have been infertile—in a sense—between the birth of my first and second baby. Each month I observed my body for signs of menstruation and was hysterical with grief when the period came. I was just as obsessed, just as depressed as any woman who cannot have children at all. It was only at the end of the year when I forced myself to be more philosophical about the whole situation that conception occurred.

The barriers to fertility can be physical, psychological or emotional. Many people find the subject difficult and embarrassing to discuss but if as a couple you wish to have your subfertility investigated, you're going to need to seek help, which means both of you discussing sensitive subjects in an open and sensible way.

Examining a woman's infertility may involve some or all of the following procedures, depending on the preferences of the center to which you are referred:
- Keeping a temperature chart during the woman's menstrual cycle to check if ovulation is occurring. The temperature rises around day 14 when you ovulate
- Examining vaginal secretions
- Discussion of frequency and type of sexual intercourse
- Surgical exploration, usually laparoscopy, in which a telescopelike instrument is passed through the abdominal wall to allow the doctor to look at your reproductive organs
- Passing a dye through your fallopian tubes which is visible on an X-ray to show up any blockages in the tubes.

Other techniques to diagnose and correct female infertility are time-consuming, lengthy and generally invasive, so they are usually deferred until your partner's sperm count and quality are checked and ruled out as a factor.

DRUG TREATMENT

The failure to ovulate or produce sufficient numbers of sperm may be corrected with drugs in some cases. The same chemicals can be used by both men and women, though the results are much better in women. First a fairly simple drug is used to stimulate ovulation in gradually increasing doses until ovulation occurs regularly. If this initial treatment fails, hormone therapy may be considered. Pregnancy results in about two-thirds of patients who receive this form of therapy and usually within a short time, about three to four months. Even with careful dosage, multiple births—particularly twins

—are hard to avoid, so you should be prepared for this. Unfortunately, approximately one in eight of these induced pregnancies may end in miscarriage.

MALE INFERTILITY

In men there are two main causes of infertility: a blockage in the tubes between the testes and the penis and inadequate production of sperm. Both of these problems require hospital investigation and laboratory tests before they can be excluded. Inadequate sperm production involves three kinds of deficiency: a low sperm count, low sperm mobility or large numbers of abnormal sperm. These characteristics have to be examined not only in the laboratory but in the woman after intercourse.

ASSISTED CONCEPTION

The ability to assist infertile couples to conceive and give birth to healthy babies has improved enormously over the past 25 years, although access to the most sophisticated techniques may be limited to a few specialist centers, and you may have to pay for private treatment. These techniques help women whose fallopian tubes are blocked, and men whose sperm counts are low or who have problems with impotence. The original technique of *in vitro* fertilization (fertilization of the egg in the laboratory followed by implantation in the woman's womb) has been refined so that the fertilized egg may be reintroduced into the womb or the fallopian tube, or sperm introduced to the egg internally so that conception occurs inside the body. It is worth facing up to the fact that only in a minority of cases do these techniques result in the desired outcome—the birth of a healthy baby—and may require more than one try at considerable expense. It is for this reason that many centers impose an upper age limit on couples they will treat.

Other forms of assisted conception are DI (donor insemination), whereby an anonymous donor's sperm are introduced into a woman's vagina or uterus, and surrogate motherhood, whereby another woman bears a child on behalf of an infertile couple.

All these methods involve complex ethical issues, and are subject to legal strictures. If assisted conception involves donor sperm or eggs, make sure you get plenty of advice and study the credentials of the clinic you are using.

HAZARDS AT WORK

If you or your partner work with certain chemicals, lead or radiation, your fertility could be affected. It is now known that certain industrial substances can damage sperm and cause malformed babies and spontaneous abortion. If you're not sure about the chemicals or other substances that you work with and how they might affect your chances of conception, ask your doctor, union representative or personnel manager. Only a relatively small number of substances have been recognized as needing a safety threshold. However, this safe level of exposure doesn't take into account how the chemicals may affect fertility. Rather than taking a chance, if one of you works with a hazardous substance, you might consider trying to change your job before conceiving a baby. If that's not possible and you can't avoid contact with doubtful substances, follow stringent safety regulations, wear protective clothing, and avoid breathing in dust or fumes or skin contact with the substance.

2

Finding out you are pregnant

There are two quite separate aspects to finding out you're pregnant. The first is about confirming your pregnancy; this can be picked up in signs from your body like nausea, having to empty your bladder more often, and dilated veins on the surface of your breasts. The other involves intellectual and emotional acceptance of your pregnancy. The first may be tinged with excitement, the second colored by feelings of ambivalence. No matter how much you've wanted to be pregnant, you may well have a mixed response to the news that you are.

A mixture of positive and negative feelings about the pregnancy is normal and nothing to feel guilty about. Uppermost in your mind will be your feelings about yourself, your partner and your relationship. Many couples find they reassess each other before accepting their new status. Eventually you'll find that becoming parents is a step forward which introduces you to a satisfying new role.

Early symptoms of pregnancy

PERHAPS THE EARLIEST symptom of pregnancy for many women is the feeling that they really are pregnant—a definite consciousness of pregnancy that I believe has as much to do with the first secretion of pregnancy hormones as anything else. These hormones affect your body in every respect, as well as your mind and the way you feel.

Another early sign is fatigue. Although some women feel energized, the majority would confess to feeling tired. It is a new kind of tiredness that they haven't felt before. Some women say that they find themselves dropping off to sleep at any time of the day; others say that they become so sleepy in the early afternoon that they have to stop what they are doing and wait for the tiredness to pass. Others are tired in the evening. Whenever it occurs, this fatigue is often uncontrollable and you just have to sleep. This condition is known as narcolepsy. I have never found a satisfactory explanation for this eccentric desire to sleep. It could well be an effect of progesterone, which reaches high levels in the blood early in pregnancy. Progesterone is a sedative in human beings with powerful tranquilizing and hypnotic effects. Progesterone also accounts for the serene and beatific look that is classically associated with pregnancy. There is another type of fatigue occurring later in pregnancy (see p. 154), which is due simply to tiredness of the body, but it rarely occurs during the first three months.

MISSED PERIOD

Within two weeks of fertilization you'll miss a period—the classic sign of pregnancy. This is called amenorrhea. While pregnancy is the commonest cause of amenorrhea, it's not the only one so don't automatically assume you're pregnant. A severe physical illness, shock, jet lag, surgery, even anxiety, are known to make a period late. Equally, it's quite common to have a light bleed after the pregnancy is established, at the time you might normally have had a period. This is why some pregnancies appear only to be eight months in length (see p. 93).

MORNING SICKNESS

Nausea, occasionally accompanied by vomiting, occurs from about week six and is often experienced as "morning sickness," though it may happen at other times of the day. It rarely continues beyond the first three months and then it gradually stops (see p. 150). It's caused by the increasing levels of hormones circulating in the blood, which can have a direct irritant effect on the lining of the stomach. One hormone, human chorionic gonadotrophin (HCG), is produced to keep up supplies of estrogen and progesterone to maintain the pregnancy. Its presence in urine confirms a pregnancy (see p. 48). The buildup of HCG roughly parallels the time of nausea, tailing off at 12–14 weeks. Hormones also cause a rapid clearing of sugar from the blood, which may result in a simultaneous feeling of hunger and sickness.

TASTES AND CRAVINGS

A change in taste and in preferences for certain foods may be one of the first signs of pregnancy, happening even before you miss a period. It's quite common to go off certain food and drink, especially fried foods, coffee and alcohol. Some women experience a metallic taste in the mouth which affects their appreciation of food. Cravings are thought to be due to the rising hormone levels and are sometimes felt during the second half of the menstrual cycle for the same reason. Don't indulge a craving for high calorie foods, which may be low in nutritional value.

FREQUENCY OF URINATION

As the uterus begins to swell, it presses on the bladder. Hormonal changes lead to differences in muscle tone, also affecting the bladder. As a result, it tries to expel even small amounts of urine, and many women notice a desire to pass urine more frequently only a week after conception. Unless there's a burning sensation or pain when you pass urine there is no need to consult your doctor about frequency of urination (micturition). Around week 12, the enlarging uterus rises up out of the pelvic cavity which reduces the pressure on the bladder for the next few months.

BREASTS

The breast changes in early pregnancy (see p. 94) are due to stimulation by progesterone. Even before you miss your first period your nipples will feel sore and your breasts will enlarge and become tender. Veins are prominent over the surface of the breasts and the creamy nodules in the nipple area (the areola) will become bigger. The nipples also start to enlarge and deepen in color.

Receiving the news

MOST OF US FEEL some ambivalence about pregnancy and parenthood and find that our feelings shift with our moods. It's absolutely normal to have mixed feelings. It would be unrealistic to imagine that your life will remain unchanged after the baby comes and it's better to think ahead. Don't feel that you're inadequate for having conflicting feelings and don't try to suppress them. It's far more sensible to acknowledge and face up to them, rather than trying to reach a point where there are no conflicts. Going through pregnancy is a phase of your emotional growth, and at the end of it you should have a better understanding and awareness of yourself.

PREGNANCY TESTS

There are various ways to confirm pregnancy. Detecting the presence of the pregnancy hormone human chorionic gonadotrophin (see p. 94) in urine is the most common test. This hormone is produced in increasing amounts in the early part of pregnancy.

Home kits

These use a urine sample and you need to follow the manufacturer's instructions since methods vary from kit to kit. Some involve adding a few drops of a substance to your urine. It is very important that you use the first urine after waking in the morning because the pregnancy hormone will be in its most concentrated form then, since nothing has been drunk or eaten for a number of hours.

Urine tests

Pass a sample of your first urine of the morning into a clean, soap-free container. Your doctor, clinic or pharmacy will arrange for the test to be done. A negative result from a urine test does not necessarily mean you are not pregnant. If the other signs persist, try again in seven days; you may have tested too early in your pregnancy. Home kits and laboratory urine tests are 95 percent reliable.

Internal examination

You may be examined internally by your doctor to confirm pregnancy although this is rarely done nowadays. Pregnancy hormones soften the consistency of your cervix and uterus and cause more blood to be directed to your pelvis, which gives the cervix the classic purplish tinge of pregnancy. Your uterus will also be slightly enlarged. To perform an internal examination, your doctor will insert two fingers into your vagina. By palpating your abdomen with the other hand, he or she can detect the general softening of the genital organs and the increase in size of the uterus. The test is not reliable before the eighth week and it doesn't harm the embryo.

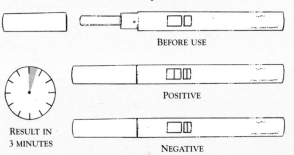

BEFORE USE

POSITIVE

RESULT IN 3 MINUTES

NEGATIVE

HOME TESTING KIT
Home kits can diagnose pregnancy two days after your missed period. In this kit, the sampler is held in your urine flow. The cap is replaced, and in three minutes the read-out on the handle gives a result.

DIFFERENT REACTIONS

The reactions to the confirmation of your pregnancy may not be what you expected. It's possible that personal circumstances change so that a pregnancy is unwelcome. A woman may resent a pregnancy taking over her body and become bitter because her active life is curtailed. Some women become depressed when they realize they are pregnant and even consider abortion.

This is painting a negative picture, more negative perhaps than the majority of women feel. However, the most important part of receiving the news that you're pregnant is for you and your partner to accept the pregnancy fully. Don't think that you can ignore it and carry on as normal just because it doesn't show for the first few weeks or months. You both have to think of your pregnancy realistically, not in a rosy glow.

HOW TO CALCULATE YOUR ESTIMATED DATE OF DELIVERY (EDD)

The average pregnancy is 266 days long measured from conception or 280 days measured from the first day of your last menstrual period (LMP). To find your EDD, find the date of your LMP in the columns of dates set in bold type; the date next to it is your EDD. You can also work it out as follows:

LMP   17.09.98
+ 9 months 17.06.99
+ 7 days   24.06.99

Remember 280 days is average and you may not be average. The possibility of your baby arriving on your EDD depends on your having regular 28-day cycles. All that doctors are prepared to say is that a normal pregnancy may be anywhere between 38 and 42 weeks.

Jan	Oct	Feb	Nov	Mar	Dec	Apr	Jan	May	Feb	June	Mar	July	Apr	Aug	May	Sept	June	Oct	July	Nov	Aug	Dec	Sept
1	8	1	8	1	6	1	6	1	5	1	8	1	7	1	8	1	8	1	8	1	8	1	7
2	9	2	9	2	7	2	7	2	6	2	9	2	8	2	9	2	9	2	9	2	9	2	8
3	10	3	10	3	8	3	8	3	7	3	10	3	9	3	10	3	10	3	10	3	10	3	9
4	11	4	11	4	9	4	9	4	8	4	11	4	10	4	11	4	11	4	11	4	11	4	10
5	12	5	12	5	10	5	10	5	9	5	12	5	11	5	12	5	12	5	12	5	12	5	11
6	13	6	13	6	11	6	11	6	10	6	13	6	12	6	13	6	13	6	13	6	13	6	12
7	14	7	14	7	12	7	12	7	11	7	14	7	13	7	14	7	14	7	14	7	14	7	13
8	15	8	15	8	13	8	13	8	12	8	15	8	14	8	15	8	15	8	15	8	15	8	14
9	16	9	16	9	14	9	14	9	13	9	16	9	15	9	16	9	16	9	16	9	16	9	15
10	17	10	17	10	15	10	15	10	14	10	17	10	16	10	17	10	17	10	17	10	17	10	16
11	18	11	18	11	16	11	16	11	15	11	18	11	17	11	18	11	18	11	18	11	18	11	17
12	19	12	19	12	17	12	17	12	16	12	19	12	18	12	19	12	19	12	19	12	19	12	18
13	20	13	20	13	18	13	18	13	17	13	20	13	19	13	20	13	20	13	20	13	20	13	19
14	21	14	21	14	19	14	19	14	18	14	21	14	20	14	21	14	21	14	21	14	21	14	20
15	22	15	22	15	20	15	20	15	19	15	22	15	21	15	22	15	22	15	22	15	22	15	21
16	23	16	23	16	21	16	21	16	20	16	23	16	22	16	23	16	23	16	23	16	23	16	22
17	24	17	24	17	22	17	22	17	21	17	24	17	23	17	24	17	24	17	24	17	24	17	23
18	25	18	25	18	23	18	23	18	22	18	25	18	24	18	25	18	25	18	25	18	25	18	24
19	26	19	26	19	24	19	24	19	23	19	26	19	25	19	26	19	26	19	26	19	26	19	25
20	27	20	27	20	25	20	25	20	24	20	27	20	26	20	27	20	27	20	27	20	27	20	26
21	28	21	28	21	26	21	26	21	25	21	28	21	27	21	28	21	28	21	28	21	28	21	27
22	29	22	29	22	27	22	27	22	26	22	29	22	28	22	29	22	29	22	29	22	29	22	28
23	30	23	30	23	28	23	28	23	27	23	30	23	29	23	30	23	30	23	30	23	30	23	29
24	31	24	1	24	29	24	29	24	28	24	31	24	30	24	31	24	1	24	31	24	31	24	30
25	1	25	2	25	30	25	30	25	1	25	1	25	1	25	1	25	2	25	1	25	1	25	1
26	2	26	3	26	31	26	31	26	2	26	2	26	2	26	2	26	3	26	2	26	2	26	2
27	3	27	4	27	1	27	1	27	3	27	3	27	3	27	3	27	4	27	3	27	3	27	3
28	4	28	5	28	2	28	2	28	4	28	4	28	4	28	4	28	5	28	4	28	4	28	4
29	5			29	3	29	3	29	5	29	5	29	5	29	5	29	6	29	5	29	5	29	5
30	6			30	4	30	4	30	6	30	6	30	6	30	6	30	7	30	6	30	6	30	6
31	7			31	5			31	7			31	7	31	7			31	(7)			31	7

49

The working woman

IN MOST COUNTRIES there are laws governing the length of time that a woman has to work in order to receive financial benefits and the conditions that her employer must meet on her return to work. Outside these laws the majority of employers are keen to cooperate with your plans for discontinuing employment before the birth and for resuming it afterwards. There is usually a statutory period of notice of maternity leave that you must give your employer; if you don't comply with this you may lose benefits, so find out about your rights as early in the pregnancy as possible. Around the end of the first trimester you should be thinking about your future work. If you wish to have your job held open for you after your maternity leave, talk to your employer to see how your plans can be accommodated.

WORKING IN PREGNANCY
Continuing to work during pregnancy helps your self-esteem and gives you a feeling of security.

WORKING DURING PREGNANCY

Unless your work involves heavy physical labor, or you work in an environment where there are harmful chemicals or fumes (see p. 45), there is no reason why you should not continue working well into pregnancy. The length of time that you will work depends on your physical fitness, the sort of job you are doing and your reason for working. One benefit of working is that it encourages everyone around you to view pregnancy as normal. As well as that, your job gives you a

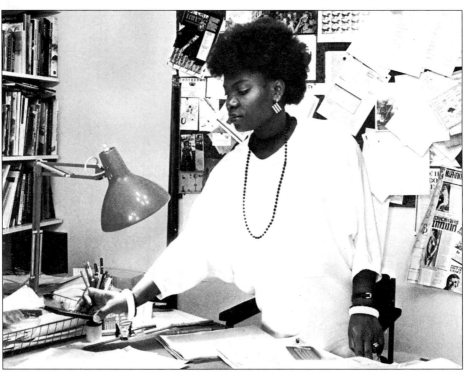

feeling of stability and security during a time when you are undergoing physical and psychological changes.

There's no hard and fast rule about when to give up work—it depends on the nature of the work you do and how physically taxing it is. Probably 32 weeks is a good time to stop as it is around this time that the greatest work load is thrown on your heart, lungs and other vital organs like the kidneys and liver, and there is a great deal of physical stress on your spine, your joints and muscles. It is a time when you should not be asking your body to do anything except rest if you feel tired. This is difficult in a job, even a sedentary one.

Whatever your job, you will have to make adjustments to your daily routine. In later pregnancy, you will lose some of your agility, and working long hours and having late nights will leave you exhausted. You will find yourself falling asleep and losing concentration. As far as household chores are concerned, let your priorities slide. Your health and that of your unborn baby are far more important than a spotless house.

TIPS FOR THE WORKING DAY

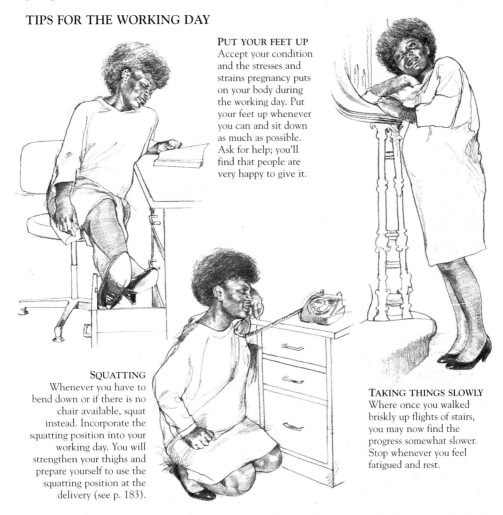

PUT YOUR FEET UP
Accept your condition and the stresses and strains pregnancy puts on your body during the working day. Put your feet up whenever you can and sit down as much as possible. Ask for help; you'll find that people are very happy to give it.

SQUATTING
Whenever you have to bend down or if there is no chair available, squat instead. Incorporate the squatting position into your working day. You will strengthen your thighs and prepare yourself to use the squatting position at the delivery (see p. 183).

TAKING THINGS SLOWLY
Where once you walked briskly up flights of stairs, you may now find the progress somewhat slower. Stop whenever you feel fatigued and rest.

BEING A WORKING MOTHER

Some women are happy to deal with pregnancy as an interruption to their work, remaining in their posts until just before going into labor, then having the baby and returning to work within the shortest time possible. They avoid the emotional dilemma of whether or not to breast or bottle feed the baby and opt for the latter. Other women would be unhappy with this decision. They want to stay with their children; anything that takes them away from their children is painful.

Women with strong maternal instincts will be concerned with not only depriving their babies of affection, but also with the sacrifices that they are making themselves. They want to enjoy their children's presence and company much of the time, and, especially while their children are young, find it distressing to leave them even for a few hours.

Nonetheless, mothers continue to work for many different reasons, which include economic necessity, the desire to be independent and self-reliant, boredom with the routine of home life, and the absolute personal need to work. As women become more able to shape their own lives, more mothers are working, and of these more and more do so simply because they enjoy it. They feel that their work greatly enriches their lives and that if it does, that will certainly help to enrich their family life.

In the past, many women thought it was their duty to ignore their own desires and serve the family; now most women feel very strongly that they have the right to take their own wishes into consideration and to make the decision to work, even if they know that it may create difficulties in the family.

Your partner's feelings should also be considered along with your own. It can lead only to unhappiness and resentment if you decide to return to work but your partner is reluctant for you to do so. If you have reason to believe that he feels this way, you must bring matters out into the open. A frank discussion with him may lead to a suitable compromise and a happy solution to your working future.

WHEN TO RETURN

If you decide that you are going to return to work after your baby is born, you might want to go back under different conditions. Discuss this with your employer during your pregnancy. There may be provision for part-time employment in your work or a phased return which allows you to be in effect a part-time worker up until one year after the baby's birth. You might like to investigate job sharing or setting up on your own in some freelance activity, which might enable you to work from home. Now is the time to think about these alternatives and plan for them.

In figuring out when you are going to restart work, you must be fair to yourself. It takes about nine months for your metabolism to return to normal after a pregnancy; parts of your body recover more quickly than others. If you menstruate three months after giving birth, this is a good sign that your ovaries are getting back to their normal cyclical routine, but not all your hormone glands will be in step with them. The muscles, ligaments and joints become more flexible and elastic to accommodate your pregnant shape and weight and need time to regain their tone and strength after the birth. Vital organs like the heart, kidneys and lungs, and your blood, gradually adjust to coping with you alone and not with you plus the baby.

BABIES AND PARENTS

A good system of childcare will be a priority and you'll have to put quite a lot of time and effort into selecting one that suits your needs. If you feel reluctant or guilty about entrusting your baby to someone else, and fear that you might be left out of your child's affections, be reassured as I was (even though only in

ADVANTAGES AND DISADVANTAGES OF BEING A WORKING MOTHER

ADVANTAGES

- increased independence
- financial rewards—the chance to raise the standard of living of your family
- career fulfillment—chance to use whatever training and qualifications you may have
- more intense interaction with your child when you are at home
- intellectual need to work—bored and lonely at home
- ability to maintain a high profile in your chosen field.

DISADVANTAGES

- sense of guilt and inadequacy because you feel you are neglecting your child
- isolation from the community
- tiredness because you are juggling two jobs at once
- great stress due to dual responsibilities and the need to be constantly planning ahead
- resentment of full-time mothers in your community
- worries about finding and keeping good child care.

retrospect) by an interesting study carried out in the last few years. When I actually was a working mother with small babies, I didn't know that this research was going on and trusted my own instinct. What I felt was that my children would know me as their mother by the biological semaphore that I sent out and that they picked up. I felt certain in my own mind, despite the presence of very loving nannies, that my children could never mistake a nanny for me, their mother. I found it difficult to pin down how they would make the distinction. I thought possibly that it would be through body smell and until they were about 18 months I made sure that they had opportunities to feel and smell my skin at feeding times and during nuzzling play.

What research showed was that babies have an even keener intelligence for singling out their parents from all other human beings than I thought. The crucial factor is the loving, interested attention that only parents can give, and a baby sorts this out from all the other stimuli. The most staggering aspect of this research is that babies need less than an hour a day of caring parental interest to thrive. The length of time spent without their parents counts far less than the quality of the time spent with them. Love isn't measured in time, love is what you put into time, no matter how short.

DUAL ROLE

Having to invest most of your free time in your family can be hard for a working mother. There's no denying that you are doing two jobs. Sometimes this is not too difficult. If you have an office job, you may have the energy to spare when you get home for bathtimes, play, story reading and sympathetic listening. However, a physical job or any job that involves caring or communication, means expending much of the sort of energy your children need during your working day.

I firmly believe that a child, especially of preschool age, has the right to expect and receive his parents' attention when they are home from work. The price of this is high. Instead of dropping into a chair or soaking in a bath when you return home, you'll have to pick up the baby and do everything else one-handed until he's asleep. When you finally fall asleep, ten to one your night will be disturbed. You don't just have to be generous of spirit, you both have to be sacrificial. There are advantages and disadvantages to being a working mother (see above); the best option for you is whatever makes you happiest. Be prepared, however, for feelings of guilt and inadequacy, but so long as you and your partner are happy, your child will do equally well whether you stay at home or go to work.

3

Choices in childbirth

Most women are aware that there are choices to be made in childbirth and, given a normal pregnancy, they can exercise many personal options. In most parts of Europe and North America, doctors and midwives form flexible teams that work towards satisfying a woman's birth preferences. You can now feel that the birth of your child is an experience over which you have control and which you are free to enjoy. Hospitals welcome the presence of your partner or someone else close to you as a birth attendant. Home births are also becoming more common and with the advent of the team midwife scheme, a doctor need no longer be present at a home birth unless complications occur.

Organizing yourself

SOME WOMEN ARE disappointed by their experience of childbirth; not the birth itself but the way it's conducted or the way they're treated. First, if you're going to have the kind of birth you want, you need to be explicit in stating your desires. Second, you have to be aware of your options. The way you can achieve this is by reading, asking questions, writing to various associations for information and guidance (see pp. 244–245), being somewhat more self-assertive than you might have been in the past and never accepting anything unless you feel entirely happy about it. Third, you are going to have to learn to communicate. It's all very well having decided in your own head what you would like to happen

but if you can't explain this to others your hopes will never be realized. Set things out on paper in a logical way so that they are clear in your own mind. If you haven't a lot of self-confidence, ask your partner or a good friend to come along for moral support when you have to face a situation that makes you anxious.

One aim of this chapter is to make it easy for you to plan the kind of childbirth you would like after assessing your own emotional and physical needs. Another aim is to give you the confidence to discuss with doctors and midwives on equal terms the options available and to state your preferences. Most hospital notes have a page for you to record your birth plan so that your wishes are available for all to see.

WHERE TO HAVE YOUR BABY

The two important elements in your choice are whether you want a medically managed or a natural childbirth and whether you want to have your baby at home or in a hospital. There are people who passionately advocate hospital high technology births, who say that this is the only way to ensure that mother and baby will be well looked after, if an emergency occurs. At the other extreme, there are natural childbirth advocates who are vehement in support of their methods. Some women feel that only in a hospital will they have the security they need. Other women wish to be surrounded by hearth and home when they give birth to their baby. You should consider the following points.

At home

For women having a normal pregnancy and a normal delivery, home birth is virtually ideal. At one time medical opinion was almost 100 percent of the view that hospital delivery was safer. However, studies have shown that women are much happier at home and it has been proved that it is at least as safe to give birth at home as in a hospital for a healthy mother and her baby.

Domino scheme

A midwife from a local team looks after you prenatally in partnership with your own family doctor or obstetrician. When you go into labor, your regular midwife, or one who is on call at the time, will meet you at the hospital and deliver you there. You're unlikely to be in the hospital more than 48 hours.

General practitioner unit

These are only available in some areas. Your doctor and a midwife look after your prenatal and postnatal care. Either the midwife or your doctor will deliver you in the unit within a hospital where the atmosphere is much less rushed than in a large maternity hospital.

Consultant maternity unit

This is obstetrician-based care within a general hospital. Most prenatal care is done in the community; however, women who may have complications attend the prenatal clinic at the hospital. In this case you may well be seen by different doctors and midwives at each visit, though now many hospitals have introduced team midwives. Several centers across the country now have birthing pools and other facilities so a woman can have the labor she prefers. For first-time mothers the support of other mothers and hospital staff during the first days is an advantage, although a busy hospital may not be restful for some. Although the emphasis in a hospital maternity unit will be on helping you to have a normal birth, it is here that you are more likely to experience so-called "high-tech" obstetric procedures, which are available if necessary.

GETTING INFORMATION

Like any other expectant animal, spend some time finding out where and how you are going to have the baby. One of the first things to do is to talk to your doctor. He or she will give you information about what is available and the various people that you might get in touch with. Your doctor will also tell you the kind of birth he or she prefers and you'll be able to assess if you're going to get on easily or if there may be conflict. This will help you to make a decision. At the same time contact your midwife. More and more women are opting for midwife-supervised births; and while it's always advisable to work with your doctor, most recognize now that a normal birth can be handled perfectly safely by a trained midwife. Your midwife will give you the addresses of the various associations to write to.

Home birth

THERE ARE ADVANTAGES to having your baby at home if your pregnancy is straightforward. You'll avoid exhausting travel to the hospital when you're already in labor, and you'll have the same midwife throughout labor and birth. Starting off breastfeeding is nearly always more successful in the home environment. The other important factor is that you lead the way in managing your labor and birth; others support you.

MOBILITY

Mobility is now recognized as being positively helpful during labor. Most women find it easier to cope with contractions if they are able to change position at will; it also helps the uterus to

work better and keeps the oxygen to the baby topped up. Although hospitals encourage mobility, many women prefer to have the freedom and privacy of moving about in their own home.

CONFIDENCE

You'll probably feel confident and relaxed because you're in a familiar place. This is a great advantage, as emotional well-being does affect the function of the uterus. You'll also avoid the possibility of cross-infection from the medical staff and other mothers and babies in the hospital. Being at

TALKING TO YOUR TODDLER
Spending time talking to your toddler about the birth will help to reassure him.

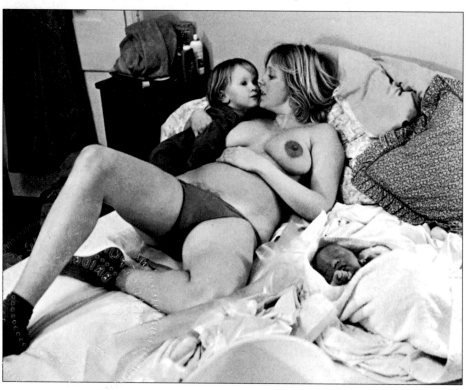

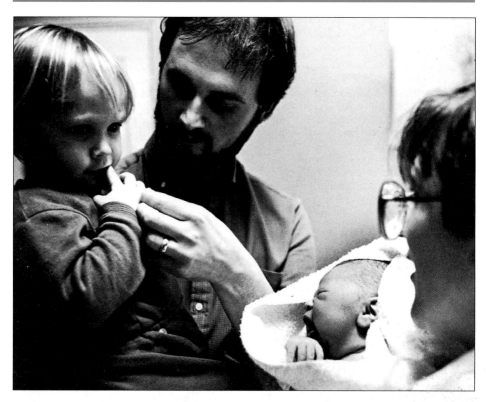

A FAMILY EVENT
If you have your baby at home the whole family will feel involved with the new baby from the start.

home will avoid many aspects of hospital care that you may find distasteful. Their absence will be a bonus.

FAMILY GROUP

By staying at home you'll avoid unhappiness caused by family separation, particularly if you have other children. Everyone can benefit from the emotional and physical bonding that develops immediately after the birth (see p. 214).

ORGANIZING A HOME BIRTH

The first step is to consult your doctor and ask if you can have maternity care from that practice. You may have to find a different doctor to look after you during pregnancy. Some doctors or even whole health authorities are unwilling to authorize home deliveries, especially in rural areas where a specialist maternity unit may be many miles away, resulting in dangerous delay if anything untoward happens during labor or birth. If there isn't a doctor in your area who does home confinements, call a relevant organization for help and advice (see pp. 244–245).

Provided there have been no problems in your health or during a previous labor, you should find a general practitioner or hospital consultant who will take responsibility for you. After you are assessed by the doctor, you can prepare for your home birth. For information about midwives and home birth resources, write to the American College of Nurse Midwives.

Hospital birth

FOR SOME WOMEN the decision to have a hospital birth is made for them because of their physical condition or their obstetric history. However, if you do need or want a hospital confinement, before you decide on a particular hospital, there are many questions that you may want to ask. Use this checklist to help you.

● Can my partner or friend stay with me all the time and after the baby is delivered?
● If I need a cesarean section, can my partner or a friend be with me?

WHY A HOSPITAL DELIVERY?

There are good reasons for having a hospital birth:

● If your medical background includes heart disease, kidney disease, high blood pressure, tuberculosis, asthma, diabetes, serious anemia, obesity or epilepsy.
● If your previous deliveries have included a stillbirth, breech presentation, a transverse or oblique lie (that is if the baby is lying sideways in the pelvis), premature labor before the 37th week, placental insufficiency where the placenta failed to nourish the baby adequately, a forceps delivery or a retained placenta.
● If the following obstetric reasons apply in your case: the baby is too big to pass through the pelvis; true postmaturity (see p. 201); you have pre-eclampsia; you are carrying twins or higher multiples; you have bleeding from the vagina late in pregnancy; the placenta is lying in the lower part of the uterus (placenta previa); there is excessive water around the baby; you are a Rhesus negative mother and tests have shown that there are sufficient antibodies in your blood to harm the baby; you have scarring of the uterus from previous cesarean sections or you are over 35 years old and it is your first baby (although this is no longer necessarily a reason for special attention if you are healthy—see p. 36).

● May I walk around during labor if everything is okay?
● May I choose the position in which I can give birth?
● Do women have their waters broken as a routine?
● What percentage of women do you induce in this hospital?
● How many women have continuous electronic fetal monitoring?
● What percentage of women have an episiotomy or a forceps delivery in this hospital?
● Can I arrange to have no drugs for pain relief in this hospital?
● When a cesarean birth is planned how many women have epidural anesthesia and how many have general anesthesia?
● Can I have as much time as I want to cuddle the baby after delivery if everything is okay?
● If I have a cesarean section can I and/or the father hold the baby afterwards?
● Can I use aromatherapy oils during labor for massage?
● Is there free visiting time?
● Is it possible to arrange a 12- or 24-hour discharge?

HOW LONG?

A fairly standard hospital stay is 48 hours, and even after a cesarean you are likely to be discharged after four days provided the incision is healing and the baby is healthy. However, it is your right to discharge yourself from the hospital, on your own responsibility, at any time. If you have adequate support and help and there are no complications with you or your baby, there is no reason why you should not go home.

YOUR PARTNER
Your partner will be with you in the hospital to encourage and reassure you throughout labor and delivery.

YOUR BIRTH PARTNER

Your partner should be closely involved in the pregnancy and birth, and he or she is the natural choice for a birth assistant. His involvement is crucial not only as support for you but also for cementing the bonds with the baby from the moment of birth. He can be the most loving and supportive "midwife." His involvement from the beginning will improve your communication in preparation for the birth, and during labor your partner is the person who gives you most attention. The medical staff are there to support the two of you. However, your birth assistant doesn't have to be your partner. You may prefer a relative or close friend instead.

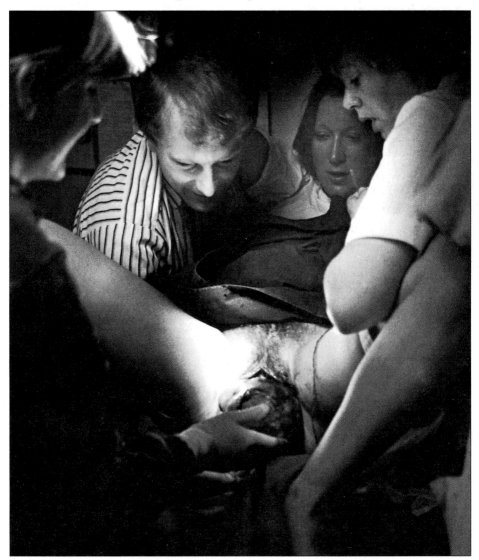

THE MIDWIFE

A midwife-supervised pregnancy and labor guarantees continuity of care, a factor that is missing from many hospital pregnancies. Whenever you attend the prenatal clinic you will see one of the team midwives so you can get to know them all during your pregnancy, and one of the team will attend you during the birth.

THE OBSTETRICIAN

Some women, however, feel cheated and nervous, even second class, if they don't have an obstetrician, as well as a midwife present at their delivery. Despite the fact that they expect nothing to go wrong, they would simply be happier in the hands of a specialist. There is yet another group of women for whom the hospital setting makes childbirth the event they expect it to be.

SENSE OF ACHIEVEMENT
After the birth, you will both feel that you have achieved something miraculous together.

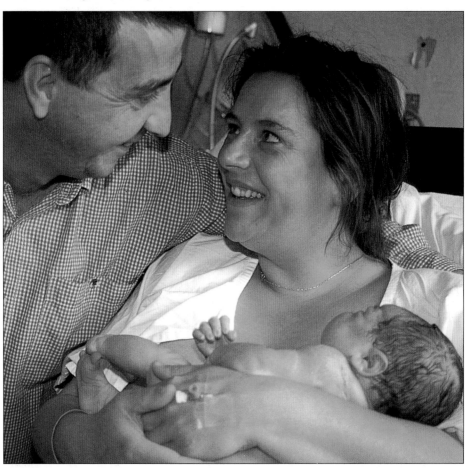

Obstetricians are busy people, and on your day of delivery he or she may not be available. You may not even see the same doctor at the prenatal clinic. If you do want to go privately, get a list of practitioners from the American College of Obstetricians and Gynecologists (see p. 244) to help you decide on the right obstetrician for you.

The natural childbirth movement

AS OBSTETRIC MEDICINE became more sophisticated, childbirth gradually came to be seen as a medical condition— something to be overseen by doctors instead of the natural, straightforward process that it really is. However from the 1960s there was a movement by women (helped by midwives) to reclaim natural childbirth. This means giving birth without fear, without unnecessary medical intervention and in a calm atmosphere. Several methods were propounded with slightly differing emphases, some of which centered on the mother, others on the baby, and still others on both. But the net result was a gradual and welcome changing of attitudes so that in the majority of hospitals the best points of the different approaches have been adopted and developed. Originally, however, there was a pure form of each method.

GRANTLY DICK-READ

In his book *Childbirth Without Fear*, first published in the 1940s, Dr. Grantly Dick-Read brought the principles of natural childbirth to public attention. His philosophy was to try to lessen and hopefully eliminate fear and tension, and the pain that resulted from these emotions, through proper education and emotional support. The Grantly Dick-Read method taught women how to cope with tension but lay strong emphasis on the fact that knowledge allays fear and prevents tension, which in turn controls pain. To help do this, he developed courses of instruction that included breathing control exercises and relaxation of muscles (see p. 143), information on what to expect in a normal situation and what women can do to help themselves. His method also taught mothers how to look for support in the form of guidance, reassurance and sympathy. Grantly Dick-Read laid great store on preparation for parenthood and childbirth itself.

PSYCHOPROPHYLAXIS

This involves training in breathing methods as a preparation for labor. The techniques were pioneered in Russia and introduced in the West by Dr. Fernand Lamaze. The Lamaze method is by far the most popular in the United States and is the basis for the teaching of the National Childbirth Trust in Britain. It encourages the woman to take responsibility for herself, to enter into partnership with her companions, friends and counselors. It greatly values team work. The woman must prepare her body throughout pregnancy with special exercises and she has to train her mind to respond automatically to each type of contraction she will feel in labor. Her partner acts as "coach" and as emotional support. He is expected to attend the course with the expectant mother and cooperate with her at home on the conditioning exercises, and he coaches, coaxes and comforts her throughout labor and delivery.

THE LEBOYER PHILOSOPHY

This relies on several basic precepts and relates more to the baby than the mother and her progress throughout labor. Dr. Frederick Leboyer in his book *Birth Without Violence* states that the newborn baby feels everything, reflecting all the emotions surrounding it—anger, anxiety, impatience and so on—and that the baby is extremely sensitive through its skin, its ears, its eyes. For that reason he believes that all stimulation to the baby should be minimized with low lights, few sounds, little handling, and with immersion in water at body heat so that the baby's entry into the world is as little different from its life in the womb as possible.

This teaching is in fact not entirely in line with the physiology of what occurs at the moment of birth for the baby. It is contact with air at a temperature different from body temperature that makes the baby take its first gulp of air to start the initial crucial function of the lungs and causes the baby's blood circulation to change from a fetal one to a mature one.

It is also simply not true to say that a baby's hearing is so sensitive that it is disturbed by noises around it. The sound of the uterine vessels within the womb are akin to a loud vacuum cleaner. Leboyer also believes that the mother is an "enemy and a monster" to the child, driving it and crushing it within the birth passage. He likens her to a torturer. Many women reasonably object to this view as it minimizes, even diminishes, the role of the mother.

Dr. Leboyer believes that the baby should not be touched by foreign materials but by human skin. The ideal place for the baby is to be laid face down on the mother's abdomen and covered by her arms. It has been proven by experiment, not Leboyer's, that this is far more efficient in preventing the baby from losing heat than overhead heaters. Research has shown that the baby is able to clear mucus from its respiratory passages more efficiently when lying face down on its mother's stomach than with a suction tube.

Leboyer suggests that the curtains and blinds in the delivery room are drawn and the lights are dimmed. Some medical authorities object to this as they say it is not possible to assess the baby's condition in a dim light.

Few centers practice the pure Leboyer method but many hospitals and community midwives practice Leboyer-based birth. It seemed to me on first reading Leboyer that all he had done was to formalize what midwives had been doing, in principle, for years. Hospitals were slower to adopt Leboyer because research has shown that Leboyer babies appear to receive no extra benefit compared to others, though many "Leboyer mothers" may feel they do.

DR. MICHEL ODENT

A French doctor named Michel Odent has advocated placing the mother in an environment which is cozy and homelike, giving her complete freedom to act as she wishes and encouraging her to reach a new level of animal consciousness where she forgets her inhibitions and returns to a rather primitive biological state. Dr. Odent believes that the high levels of endorphins, the body's natural narcotics, should be allowed to have full rein in the mother's body. He logically argues that if a woman is given painkillers and analgesics her endorphins are cut off, thus depriving her of the benefit of natural pain relief.

Dr. Odent's clinic in Pithiviers, France, where he pioneered his natural childbirth techniques, became a center for those who wished to change opinions and practices in childbirth. Dr. Odent believes that during labor there should be music, soft furnishings, and a relaxed atmosphere. A woman who goes into labor should be allowed to sit, walk, stand, eat and drink, and do whatever she wants. Women should not be interfered with in any way and can take up whatever position is most comfortable at any stage of the labor. Left to their own devices many women take up a position on all fours which seems to help the pain. Later on in birth many stand up or semi-squat so that the force of gravity can help them, a natural thing to do, which most primitive tribes practice. Odent encourages the supported squatting position where he, or the woman's partner, stands behind her, takes her weight underneath her armpits and upper arms and allows her to bend her knees and place her weight on her partner's arms.

Dr. Odent believes that birthing pools, which he now uses for many home water births, should be primarily viewed as a means of pain relief. The birth itself does not need to be underwater, though Dr. Odent is quite happy to deliver the baby into the water of the bath if that is what happens. There seems to be no proof that an underwater birth is dangerous to the baby so long as the head is lifted out of the water immediately.

Dr. Odent's methods have always had low rates of episiotomy, forceps and cesarean section. The supported squat position is the one which prevents severe perineal tears during delivery. Because the mother has been in an upright position when the baby emerges she remains sitting upright with the cord still intact and the baby in her lap. The baby immediately smells the mother's skin and it is thought that this is important to the baby in establishing breastfeeding. Within a few seconds most mothers instinctively lift the baby up and place it at the breast. No partner needs to be told to encircle the mother and the baby with his own body and arms. Each will do what comes naturally in these very personal moments.

YOGA-BASED METHODS

This is not just for those who already practice yoga. During birth a woman should concentrate her awareness on being totally at one with what is happening to her. Through yogic methods she is able to control her awareness according to her capacity and tolerance so at some times she is able to distract herself from the contractions and at others be totally involved in them. She may use meditation and chanting with the support of yoga groups' spiritual participation. Practitioners in the yogic methods believe that a woman can handle childbirth in a mature and serene way. Yogic childbirth education helps in the belief that a woman has the ability to create or destroy her own pain and joy during birth.

Nursing and medical procedures

ONE OF THE MOST WELCOME outcomes of the natural childbirth movement has been the shift in emphasis back to the mother and her needs in hospital births. Practices that were once routine such as enemas and shaving pubic hair are no longer performed, and mothers are not confined to bed; in fact even epidurals allow some mobility. Midwives and hospital staff constantly review procedures and guidelines. They have accepted wholeheartedly the findings of much research from around the world that has proved the efficacy of mobility during labor.

An excellent study done in Latin America has shown that in a group of mothers having their first baby, the length of labor in those who were allowed to move around as they wanted to was only two-thirds that of the women who were confined to bed. When all mothers were considered, the mobile group were 25 percent quicker in producing their babies than those who did not move around.

The study also found that 95 percent of mothers who are left to themselves prefer to be upright and are more comfortable when upright. When mothers spend time in different positions in labor they report less pain and greater comfort when sitting, standing, kneeling or squatting.

The study concluded that in normal spontaneous labor, women who are allowed to assume a vertical position have an easier progress through labor, shorten its duration and have less discomfort and pain. In the light of all this, no midwife would now deny women who are having normal labors the right to choose the position or positions that they find most comfortable during the first and second stages of labor, since this is likely to be the most advantageous position for them in terms of their pelvic shape and the position of the baby. Lying on the back for delivery is now sometimes discouraged for the reasons given below.

POSITIONS FOR DELIVERY

Before the end of the seventeenth century when labor rooms were solely the province of women, no one considered that the normal behavior of a woman in childbirth should be interfered with. She was allowed to move about as she wanted, take up any position that she felt was comfortable, eat and drink as she wished and assume her chosen position for delivering the baby. Then doctors invaded the delivery room and at that time all doctors were men. A doctor at the French royal court proposed that women should lie on their backs in preference to using upright positions and birthing stools to make vaginal examinations and obstetric maneuvers easier, not because it might benefit the mother or the baby.

It is natural for a woman to take up a semivertical position for delivery of the baby, not just because it's comfortable but because it is mechanically most efficient. When she is upright the uterine contractions are aiming downwards, pushing the baby out towards the floor. When a woman pushes she strains downwards in the same direction and most importantly the force of gravity helps the birth too.

When a woman lies on her back, the uterine contractions push the baby into the bed and not down the birth canal so the added advantage of the force of gravity is lost. The result is that the recumbent woman has to push her baby up and against the force of gravity. This not only prolongs labor but makes it more likely that complications may occur (see below left).

In the past, many hospital units put women into the "lithotomy position" in which a woman lies on her back with her legs up and her ankles supported by stirrups. This is never used for normal deliveries, although if you have a forceps or ventouse delivery (see pp. 209 and 213) your legs may be put in stirrups to allow the doctor a good view to pull the baby out in a straight line. However, even in these circumstances you will be propped up with pillows, not lying flat.

DISADVANTAGES OF LYING ON YOUR BACK FOR DELIVERY

If you lie on your back:
- your blood pressure may drop, thus reducing the amount of blood and oxygen to the baby
- pain is greater in this position than in a vertical one
- there is a greater need for an episiotomy
- there is an increased chance of a forceps delivery
- it inhibits spontaneous delivery of the placenta
- there is a greater possibility of low back strain in this position.

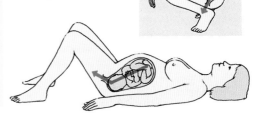

DELIVERY POSITION
It is more efficient to give birth in a semivertical position. The force of gravity helps to push the baby down and out rather than into the bed, which happens if you are lying flat on your back.

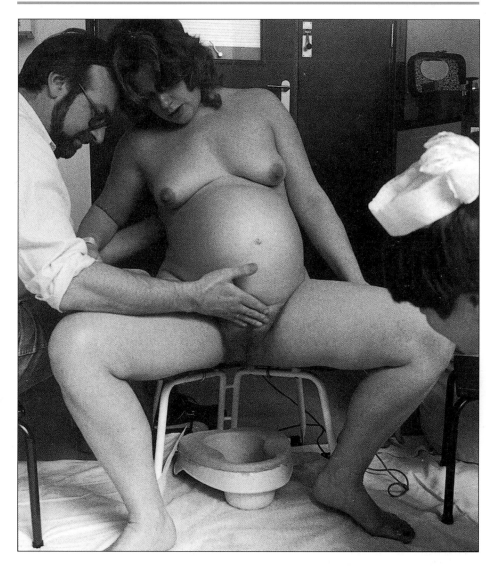

BIRTHING STOOL
A birthing stool allows you to give birth in a vertical position so that the force of gravity can help you to push the baby out.

FOOD AND DRINK

During labor the stomach seems to close down, and any food eaten during this time may be vomited up. For this reason it is a good idea to have something light and easily digestible to eat very early in labor while you are still at home to give you reserves of energy. Take glucose tablets into the delivery room with you in case you have a sudden demand for energy.

Doctors and midwives are reluctant to allow you to eat or drink during labor in case you need an emergency general anesthetic if there are problems.

However, I don't believe that this is a good enough reason to withhold food from all women—it should only be an option for those who are definitely at risk of needing a surgical procedure.

Most women in labor don't want to eat but most do require fluids, particularly as labor advances and fluids are lost through sweating, so water should be given, in my opinion, whenever it is requested. If a mother starts to become dehydrated during labor, an intravenous drip may have to be set up to administer glucose solution directly to the mother's bloodstream, bypassing the stomach and thereby increasing the medical intervention in her labor.

THE DELIVERY ROOM

In most hospitals nowadays you will go through your labor and deliver your baby in the same room. The only time you are likely to be moved is if you have to have an emergency cesarean—some units prefer to do this in a designated operating room. At your prenatal clinic ask about the delivery rooms. Most hospital-based prenatal classes will include a tour of the delivery suite and postnatal wards; try to take advantage of this so you know what to expect.

Most delivery rooms now have soft lighting, pictures on the walls and pleasant, homely soft furnishings. There will be a bed (not an old-fashioned delivery table), but you may also be able to use a mat on the floor or a beanbag for back support. Some of the more progressive units make birthing pools available as an aid to pain relief. If there is no pool in the hospital you are going to, and there is an appropriate room and the staff are amenable, it may be possible for you to rent one.

You can also use aromatherapy during labor: to perfume the birthing pool, in massage oil and on your pillow. Ask what is available in your hospital and what you can bring with you to make your labor as comfortable as possible. You'll be able to deliver almost exactly as if you are at home but with medical facilities on tap should either you or your baby need them.

Choosing how to feed

THE MOST IMPORTANT ASPECT of infant feeding is feeding the infant. Most babies thrive whether they are breast or bottle fed. Given that as a basis (and in your worst moments remind yourself of this as your overriding priority), think about the other considerations.

In order to make a choice and exercise an option you have to be aware of the pros and cons of breast and bottle feeding or a combination of both. You must bear in mind your own preferences because feeding will be most successful if you are happy with the method you have chosen. And you must also think about what is best for your baby. Although bottle feeding is convenient, there's little doubt that where the baby's well-being is concerned, breastfeeding is superior.

ADVANTAGES OF BREASTFEEDING

● A good reason for breastfeeding is that it's the natural thing to do. Most women have a natural urge to breastfeed, and there are very few women who are not physically equipped to breastfeed. No matter how small the breasts, they will be able to produce enough milk to feed and sustain the baby. Even women whose nipples are inverted can, with early diagnosis, breastfeed their babies (see p. 95).
● It's natural for a mother to feel proud that her baby is being fed on food that she provides and it's natural to crave the physical nearness and pleasure and to know that you are helping a close relationship to develop between you and your child.

• Breastfed babies are less liable to illness than bottle-fed ones. There are fewer cases of gastroenteritis, chest infection and measles. All the mother's antibodies to bacterial and viral infections are present in the colostrum, the first milk made by the breasts that is present in the breasts from the fifth month of pregnancy. In the first few days of life, therefore, when the baby is taking only the high-protein colostrum, she is living under the umbrella of her mother's antibodies. They have a protective effect in the intestine but also, as they're absorbed straight into the baby's system unchanged, they form an important part of the baby's own protection against infections. Take the example of a mother who has antibodies to poliomyelitis in her own body. Because those antibodies appear in her colostrum, it's not possible to infect her baby with the poliomyelitis virus while she's being wholly breastfed. The antibodies in the baby's gut will kill the virus before it can do any harm. Besides that, human milk is antibacterial because it contains substances that destroy bacteria. Even though these substances are present in cow's milk, a bottle-fed baby is not protected in the same way because the antibodies are inactivated when the cow's milk is heated.

• Human breast milk is the best source of food for a human baby; it has just the right amount of minerals and proteins. Cow's milk, which is for calves, has a higher percentage of protein and a high content of casein, which is the least digestible part of it and is passed out in the stool in the form of curds.

• Human milk contains just the right amount of sodium (salt) for a newborn baby. This is important because the immature kidneys of the infant are unable to deal with high levels of sodium in the blood. Cow's milk contains more sodium than human milk.

• While human milk and cow's milk contain the same amount of fat, the droplets in human milk are smaller and more digestible. Breast milk fat is high in polyunsaturates and low in cholesterol, and it may therefore protect against heart disease in later life. Breast milk also contains more sugar (lactose) than cow's milk and the mineral and vitamin content is different.

• Breastfeeding is good for the figure. Research has shown that a woman loses most of the fat she's accumulated during pregnancy if she breastfeeds. If you don't feed your baby yourself, you'll probably have more difficulty returning to your pre-pregnancy weight.

• It's a common fallacy that the breasts lose their shape and firmness through breastfeeding. This is not so. The changes that occur in the breasts are a consequence of becoming pregnant, not of producing milk or feeding your baby.

• Breastfeeding also has the advantage that it releases the hormone oxytocin which encourages the uterus to shrink to its nonpregnant size, hastening the return to normal of the pelvis and your waistline.

• The sheer convenience of breastfeeding also mustn't be ignored. Milk is always available for the baby at any time of the day or night, it doesn't have to be warmed up, there's no expensive equipment to buy and keep sterile, and it's free.

• Bonding occurs between mother and baby quite automatically if you breastfeed. When a baby is at the breast, her face is close to her mother's face—about 8–10 in. (20–25 cm)—and even a newborn baby can focus at this distance (see p. 214). The act of making eye contact and smiling at your baby as she sucks, helps to create a physical and emotional bond between mother and baby which is hardly ever broken for the rest of their lives.

PROBLEMS OF BREASTFEEDING

One of the often quoted disadvantages of breastfeeding is that it curtails social activity. This need not necessarily be so. During the early weeks babies are very portable and you can take your baby with you when you go out. Although feeding in public places can still cause raised eyebrows, it's easy to feed discreetly, and some stores, restaurants, train terminals and airports now have designated baby-feeding areas.

● If you don't want to take your baby with you, you can take off sufficient milk with a breast pump (see p. 236) to serve the baby's needs while you're away from her. You can bottle your own breast milk in sterile bottles and store them in the fridge or freezer and your babysitter can give the bottle to your baby later on your behalf. Remember, even if you only feed your

baby for two weeks, that's better than not breastfeeding at all and it will give your baby a flying start in life. Incidentally, one of the advantages of expressing some of your milk into bottles is that your partner can then become involved with the feeding routine too.

BOTTLE FEEDING

● As there are no real arguments against breastfeeding, it is also true to say that there are no arguments in favor of bottle

---

BREASTFEEDING AFTER A CESAREAN

You may fear if you are advised to have a cesarean delivery, that it will be too uncomfortable to breastfeed in the first weeks after the birth, so you may feel you should opt to bottle feed from the start. However, your midwife or obstetric physiotherapist will show you comfortable positions for breastfeeding so that the baby does not press against your wound. One way

is to lay your baby on pillows on your lap, or to tuck your baby's body under your arm with her head close to your breast. Alternatively you can lay your baby down next to you as shown below.

LYING DOWN TO BREASTFEED
You can lay your baby next to you while you lie down so she can feed from your lower breast. This is also a good way to breastfeed in bed at night.

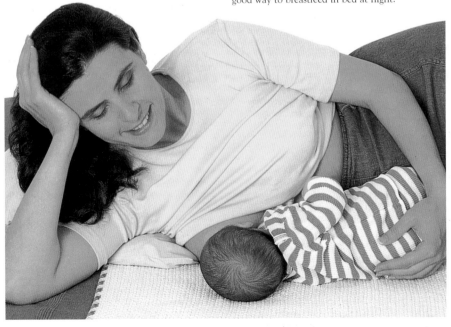

feeding. However, for you in your particular circumstances with your particular predilections, breastfeeding may not be a feasible or workable alternative, in which case bottle feeding will be your choice. If it is, don't feel that your child is getting second best.

• Babies thrive and are perfectly happy being bottle fed, and always remember that your baby needs your love and care more than she needs your breast milk. Bottle feeding, love and attention are an excellent option for any baby.

• There will be certain mothers who don't have any option but to bottle feed. These are women who may be taking drugs in the long term for a medical condition, such as epilepsy which needs barbiturates to keep it under control, or chronic depression for which antidepressants are prescribed. You may become seriously ill and need admission to a hospital. If physically you're not in a fit state to breastfeed, then you should not. If you have to take any medicines regularly, discuss with your doctor whether they are passed on to your baby in breast milk and what the possible effects will be on breastfeeding and your baby. Quite often it's possible for nursing mothers to change to safer drugs.

• Some handicapped babies, or babies with physical abnormalities such as cleft palate or deformity of the jaw and mouth, may not be able to suck the breast successfully and will have to be spoon or bottle fed.

• If you think your milk supply is inadequate and the baby is failing to thrive, consult your midwife or a breastfeeding counselor before opting to bottle feed. Your own nutrition and physical fitness do have a bearing on successful breastfeeding so you need to pay attention to getting a balanced diet (see p. 108).

• Some women have a strong physical revulsion against breastfeeding and find it a tiresome chore. A woman who feels revulsion very strongly will be under stress, and this may interfere both with milk production and milk flow. If you feel that your baby is not getting enough, these negative messages will also reinforce your dislike of breastfeeding. If this happens to you, do try to talk over your feelings before the birth of your baby with a sympathetic friend or midwife and do involve your baby's father.

• One of the main advantages of bottle feeding is that your partner can be equally involved in feeding your baby from the outset, which allows him or her to create a close, nurturing bond with the baby. It also means that you can work out a shared feeding schedule which gives you each enough time for rest, for unbroken sleep and time off for yourselves.

• One of the questionable advantages of bottle feeding is that babies sleep longer between feeds during the first weeks (although this is by no means always the case). This longer sleeping period could be because the casein content of cow's milk is higher than that of human milk and takes longer to digest.

• With bottle feeding, you can see exactly how much milk your baby has taken, which can be most reassuring.

PROBLEMS WITH BOTTLE FEEDING

• The spit-up from a bottle-fed baby has an unpleasant smell, as do the stools.

• Some babies are allergic to the alien protein in cow's milk. There are soya substitutes for babies with allergies; nursing mothers in families with a history of eczema or asthma are advised to breastfeed or use these substitutes.

• The sterilization of bottle-feeding equipment and the careful preparation of feeds are time-consuming compared to the accessibility of breast milk.

• Bottle-fed babies are more prone to gastric infections than breastfed babies, who receive some protection from their mothers' milk.

• The cost of formula milk, bottles, nipples and sterilizing equipment is substantial, whereas breastfeeding is free and is always available.

4

Prenatal care

Prenatal care is the key to healthy mothers, happy pregnancies and thriving babies and its importance can't be overemphasized. It's now accepted by most doctors that the one way in which we can improve the statistics on childbirth is through early and vigorous prenatal care. For most women, attendance at prenatal clinics, whether in the hospital or a local surgery, is smooth and happy. By talking to other mothers and to doctors and midwives, you can find out more about pregnancy and birth, which should help to reassure you and make you feel more confident about forthcoming events. Much of the prenatal care is routine, but at the clinic you can ask questions and explore the different circumstances in which you can have your baby so that you can plan ahead to get the kind of birth you want.

Going to the doctor

AS SOON AS YOU SUSPECT or know that you are pregnant, make an appointment to go to see your doctor. He or she will want to know the date of the first day of your last menstrual period (LMP) as it is from this day that the pregnancy is measured. Depending on how far your pregnancy is advanced, your doctor will perform some kind of pregnancy test— either a urine test (see p. 48) or a blood test if you have missed at least one menstrual period. He or she may want to confirm the pregnancy even if you have already used a home kit yourself and know that you're definitely pregnant.

The first visit to your doctor is important not just for confirmation of the pregnancy. It's at this first meeting that you can discuss in general terms the options for birth (see pp. 54–69), so give the subject some thought before you go along, for example whether you would like a home or hospital birth. Your preferences may conflict with your doctor's desire to stick to routines and procedures that he or she is used to and is reluctant to change, particularly with regard to home births. It's helpful for your partner to accompany you to this first appointment so you can discuss these issues together and iron out any difficulties from the start.

If you are over 35 or you have some history of genetic disorders in the family, your doctor may refer you for a chorionic biopsy (see p. 79). This procedure should be done around weeks 10–12, so visit your doctor early to get a letter of referral.

Use your doctor as a source of information: ask for a list of recommended books to read and pamphlets to send off for. If your own doctor does not specialize in obstetrics, he or she may pass you on to another member of the practice, or you may even be referred to a neighboring practice where they undertake prenatal care and home confinement if this is what you want.

The other option is to attend the local hospital or the hospital of your choice depending on your area, in which case you will be looked after by the medical staff at the hospital and not by your own doctor.

Prenatal clinics

AFTER CONFIRMATION of the pregnancy your doctor will make arrangements for your prenatal care. This will depend upon the sort of birth you want. Some prenatal care is undertaken at specialist prenatal clinics, whether they are attached to health centers or large regional hospitals. Attending a prenatal clinic in a large hospital may sometimes mean a long wait.

However, you'll probably have to go to a hospital clinic more than once every month only if there is a specific reason for you to be examined by an obstetrician, such as high blood pressure, which may be a sign of pre-eclampsia (see p. 162), or if you have some underlying medical condition such as diabetes.

PRENATAL CLASSES
You can find out about prenatal classes at your clinic. Attending classes as a couple can be enjoyable as well as helpful; you'll meet other couples whose pregnancies are at the same stage as yours and you can compare notes with them.

COPING AT THE CLINIC

If you feel like a case number, bored and frustrated by lengthy procedures at the hospital prenatal clinic, try to make the best of your time there by preparing in the following ways:

● take along a friend or a good book or some knitting or needlework
● take a small snack in case the hospital refreshment trolley doesn't come by while you're there or it's difficult for you to get to the cafeteria
● make notes of all the questions you want to ask and note any worries even if you're not sure if they're linked to your pregnancy or not
● try to get your other children cared for while you go to the clinic; they may get bored and make you nervous.

ROUTINE PRENATAL TESTS

NAME	PURPOSE	SIGNIFICANCE
HEIGHT 1st visit	To assess size of pelvis and pelvic outlet.	Very short height can suggest a small pelvic outlet and consequently maybe a difficult delivery.
WEIGHT every visit	To check that weight gain or loss is not excessive.	Excessive weight gain may put undue strain on the heart. Sudden weight gain may indicate pre-eclampsia (see p. 162).
BREASTS 1st visit unless there is a problem	Check for lumps and condition of nipples.	If nipples are retracted and you wish to breastfeed, you may be advised to wear a breast shield (see p. 95), do gentle exercises on the nipples or just wait and see. They may correct themselves during the pregnancy.
HEART, LUNGS, HAIR, EYES, TEETH, NAILS 1st visit	To check on your general physical health.	You may need some special attention and dietary supplements (see p. 113) or just general advice on diet. Dental visits will be encouraged.
LEGS AND HANDS occasionally	To look for varicose veins and any swelling (edema) in the ankles, hands or fingers.	Cases of extreme puffiness can be a sign of pre-eclampsia (see p. 162). Advice on what to do about varicose veins will be given (see p. 154).
URINE (MSU) 1st visit	To test for kidney infection. After cleaning the vulva with sterile pads, you pass a sample of urine into a sterile container. Allow the first drops to go into the toilet bowl and collect the midstream urine (MSU) only.	An existing kidney infection you may not know you have can develop into a serious condition in pregnancy. You will be treated with antibiotics.
URINE every visit	1 Tests for protein in case your kidneys aren't coping well. 2 Tests for the presence of sugar; if sugar is found repeatedly, you may have diabetes. 3 Tests for ketones.	1 Protein in urine late in pregnancy is a sign of pre-eclampsia (see p. 162). Bed rest will probably be prescribed. 2 Pregnancy can unmask diabetes (see p. 157), which must be treated and stabilized. It may go away after delivery only to return in later pregnancies. 3 Presence of ketones indicates that the body is short of sugar. This may be a sign of diabetes—if so, further tests will be made to confirm it and you will be treated accordingly. Alternatively you may simply not be eating enough and you'll be given advice on an adequate diet.
FETAL HEART-BEAT after week 14	To confirm that the fetus is alive and that the heart and heart rate are normal.	If the midwife listens to your baby's heart with a Doppler (this listens to the fetal heart with ultrasound vibrations), the sound of the beat will be amplified and you will be able to hear it too.

NAME	PURPOSE	SIGNIFICANCE
ABDOMINAL PALPATION sometimes	To assess the height of the fundus (the top of the uterus—see p. 97), and the size and position of the fetus.	Gives a guide to the length of the pregnancy and the lie of the fetus in the womb. Palpation after 36 weeks indicates the lie of the fetus. This may indicate whether the baby is in the breech position (see p. 204).
BLOOD PRESSURE every visit	This is the measurement of the pressure at which the heart is pumping blood through your body. The test is done to assess if it is normal or not. The reading is made up of two numbers: the top one is the systolic pressure, when the heart contracts, pushes out blood and "beats." This can be heard when the arm band is tightened; the bottom one is the diastolic pressure, the resting pressure between heartbeats. A normal BP is 120/70.	Hypertension (high blood pressure) can indicate a number of problems, including pre-eclampsia (see p. 162). Constant checks mean it can be kept under control if it suddenly rises, e.g., above 140/90. May mean bed rest in the hospital if it rises. Any rise in the lower or diastolic figure is cause for concern.
BLOOD TESTS 1st visit and once during 3rd trimester	1 To find your major blood group: A, B, AB or O. 2 To find your Rhesus blood group. 3 To find your hemoglobin level (repeated test). This is a measure of the oxygen-carrying substances in your red blood cells. Normal levels, measured in gm, are between 12 and 14 gm. 4 Alpha-fetoprotein levels—a special test at 16 weeks. 5 To detect the presence of German measles antibodies. 6 VDRL, Kahn or Wasserman tests for the presence of syphilis. 7 To detect or confirm sickle cell disease and thalassemia, both forms of anemia mainly found in dark-skinned people and those from the Mediterranean region. 8 To check whether the mother is HIV positive (done by consent).	1 Blood group needed in case of an emergency transfusion. 2 In case of Rhesus incompatibility (see p. 162). 3 During pregnancy your hemoglobin level may drop, because pregnant women have more circulating blood (see p. 98), but if it goes below 12–15 gm/dl, treatment for anemia (see p. 156) will be given. Iron and folic acid supplements will raise the hemoglobin level so that more oxygen can be carried to the baby. 4 See p. 77. 5 To find out whether or not you have immunity to rubella; if not you will be warned not to come into contact with German measles during your pregnancy (see p. 36). 6 If you unknowingly have this sexually transmitted infection, it is essential to treat it before week 20 of your pregnancy; after this time it can be passed to the baby. 7 Can affect the baby and the pregnancy. If either condition is found and you were not already aware of it, you will be given folic acid supplements. 8 Antibodies can cross the placenta to the baby. The baby will probably be delivered by cesarean.

THE FIRST VISIT

The purpose of your first visit to the prenatal clinic at around 12 weeks is to give information to the staff so that they can judge whether or not your pregnancy and delivery will be normal. If you want to have a home delivery, you will be asked about the social and domestic side of your life to assess whether your circumstances are suitable for home delivery.

The staff will also run certain tests on you to see if you are healthy (see p. 72); for instance, taking your blood pressure, collecting a sample of your blood and testing your urine. Blood and urine tests

YOUR PRENATAL FILE

At the initial interview you will be asked some or all of the following questions about your relevant medical and past obstetric history:

● your name, age, race, date and place of birth, and your date of marriage, if any, and the name of your next of kin
● about your childhood illnesses, and whether or not you have ever been in hospital or had any serious disease or any surgical operations
● if any illnesses run in your family or your partner's family
● whether there are twins in either family
● whether you used contraceptives, if so what sort and when you stopped
● about your menstrual history: when your periods first started, how long your average cycle is, how many days you bleed and the date of the first day of your last menstrual period
● whether you have any pregnancy symptoms and what your general state of health is like
● about the births of any other children you may have, or any miscarriages
● whether you are taking any prescription medicines or suffer from any allergies
● what work you and your partner do and whether you are still working.

may have to be sent away to a laboratory and the results will come back later and be available at your next visit.

Ask questions, too. It's important for you to gain confidence in your pregnancy by expressing any concerns. It isn't essential now at the first visit, but it's as well to discuss your preferences for pain relief during the labor, whether you want an early discharge, and what course of action you want if the baby is overdue. Your file and notes will be made available to you.

At the end of the visit you may be given iron tablets (see p. 113) and you can ask to see a dietitian if you need information about diet and nutrition. You will probably attend the prenatal clinic every four to six weeks up to 36 weeks, and thereafter every one to two weeks. Check-ups are more flexible than they used to be, and their frequency will depend on your health and the health of your baby.

When you enroll at a prenatal clinic you'll be told about the prenatal classes and will be given details of where they're held and at what time.

THE MEDICAL STAFF

● The midwife is a nurse with special training in the care of normal pregnant women and the delivery of their babies. If all goes well a midwife will deliver your baby whether at home or in a hospital. Midwives also work in the community and once you return home after delivery, you might be visited by a midwife after the birth.
● Your family doctor may be responsible for part of your prenatal care. He or she may attend your delivery at home, although family doctors do not routinely attend home births; if all is well they are happy to leave it to the midwife.
● The obstetrician is the hospital doctor who specializes in pregnancy and birth, and he or she heads the team of midwives, nurses and other doctors who provide your prenatal care and deliver your baby. The consultant obstetrician usually attends only the difficult births.

THE CLINIC

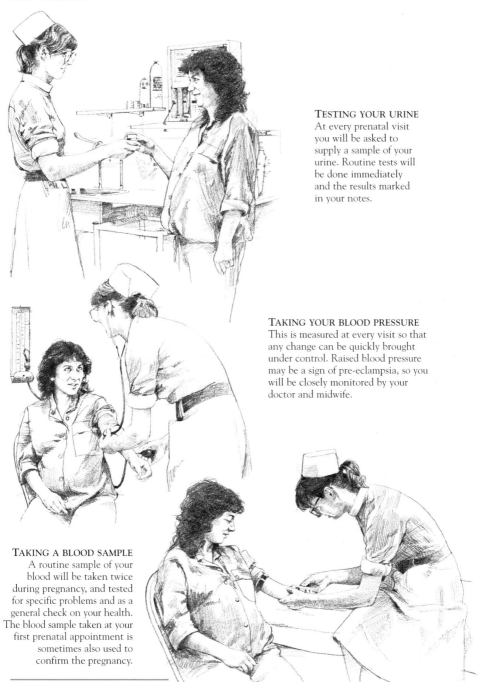

TESTING YOUR URINE
At every prenatal visit you will be asked to supply a sample of your urine. Routine tests will be done immediately and the results marked in your notes.

TAKING YOUR BLOOD PRESSURE
This is measured at every visit so that any change can be quickly brought under control. Raised blood pressure may be a sign of pre-eclampsia, so you will be closely monitored by your doctor and midwife.

TAKING A BLOOD SAMPLE
A routine sample of your blood will be taken twice during pregnancy, and tested for specific problems and as a general check on your health. The blood sample taken at your first prenatal appointment is sometimes also used to confirm the pregnancy.

UNDERSTANDING YOUR HOSPITAL NOTES

At your first prenatal visit you will be given your hospital notes. At every visit your doctor or midwife will record on them details of the routine tests and the progress of the pregnancy. Take your copies of the notes with you to every clinic. Keep them with you if you go out of your area—if you should need medical attention, all the information will be at hand. Most of the abbreviations are explained below.

NAD/nil/✓	Nothing abnormal discovered in urine
Alb	Albumin in urine (a name for one of the proteins found in urine)
BP	Blood pressure
FHH/NH	Fetal heart heard or not heard
FH	Fetal heart
FMF	Fetal movements felt
Ceph.	Cephalic, the baby is head down
Vx	Vertex, the baby is head down
Br.	Breech, the baby is bottom down
LMP	Last menstrual period
EDD/EDC	Estimated date of delivery or confinement
Hb	Hemoglobin levels to check for anemia
Eng/E	Engaged, the baby's head has dropped into the pelvis ready for birth
NE	Not engaged
Para O	Woman has no other children
Para 1 (etc)	Woman has one child
Fe	Iron has been prescribed
TCA	To come again
PET	Pre-eclamptic toxemia
Long L	Longitudinal lie, the baby is parallel to your spine in the womb
Height of fundus	The height of the top of the uterus. The baby pushes this up as it grows and often the height is used to estimate the length of the pregnancy. Some clinics measure the height of the fundus (from the top of the pubic bone to the top of the uterus) with a tape measure. This figure is usually roughly the same as the pregnancy in weeks.
Relation of PP to brim	This is the brim of your pelvis. The presenting part (PP) of the baby to the brim in the later stages of your pregnancy will be the part in your cervix ready to be born first.
Oed.	Oedema
RSA	Right sacrum anterior—the most common breech position
AFP	Alpha fetoprotein
CS	Cesarean section
H/T	Hypertension
MSU	Midstream urine sample
Primigravida	First pregnancy
Multigravida	More than one pregnancy
VE	Vaginal examination

THE LIE OF THE BABY
Certain abbreviations describe the way the baby is lying in the womb (see p. 173 and 204). They refer to the position of the crown of the baby's head (occiput) in relation to your body; that is whether on the right or the left, to the front (anterior) or back (posterior).

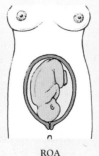
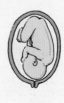
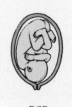

ROA   LOA   ROP   LOP

THE OLDER WOMAN

Nowadays the age of the mother is much less important than her medical history, diet and lifestyle (see p. 34). However, if you're over 35, you may still be asked extra questions at your first prenatal appointment. Once all the questions are answered, any tests performed (see below), and you're found to be generally fit and well, your care will be no different from that of younger women.

PARENTCRAFT CLASSES

First-time parents can gain confidence and information from these classes. They should ideally cover an understanding of pregnancy and birth; techniques of relaxation and breathing to prepare for labor; and caring for a small baby. Hospital-run classes will help you understand the procedures in that hospital and you will be able to see the delivery suite and postnatal wards.

Special tests

THERE ARE A NUMBER of tests available to check for any potential physical or chromosomal abnormality in the fetus. The tests include alpha fetoprotein (AFP) screening or the triple test, and invasive techniques such as amniocentesis or chorionic villus sampling (CVS). None of the tests detailed here is compulsory and a few, such as the triple test, are only available at specialist centers. Discuss them with your midwife or doctor.

AFP SCREENING

Alpha fetoprotein (AFP) is a substance found in the blood of a pregnant woman that varies in level throughout the pregnancy. Between 16 and 18 weeks the levels are usually low, so if your blood is examined for AFP at this time, and the levels are raised, you could be carrying a baby with a neural tube defect such as spina bifida, or other abnormalities of brain development. However, this test has been virtually superseded by ultrasound scans to check nuchal tube translucency (see page 79).

Raised AFP levels in the blood are not, however, conclusive evidence of neural tube defect. In addition, AFP levels may be raised with a twin pregnancy and may also rise as pregnancy progresses. If a blood test indicates raised levels, an ultrasound scan will be taken to check for twins or to confirm your dates in case the pregnancy is more advanced than you thought. A further blood test will then be taken. Only if these checks prove positive and if corroboration is needed will amniocentesis be contemplated because to be certain, alpha fetoprotein must also be found in abnormal quantities in the amniotic fluid. Minor neural tube defects such as a small hairy mole at the bottom of the spine are quite common.

Lower than normal levels of AFP indicate the risk of Down's syndrome; in this case amniocentesis will be offered.

TRIPLE TEST

The triple test is another maternal serum screening test, also known as the Bart's triple test, the Leeds test, the Biomark, or the Beta Triple. An extension of the AFP test, it also measures other hormones present in the woman's blood, such as estriol and human chorionic gonadotrophin. The test is done in the 16th week of pregnancy, and the results take about two weeks to come through. The results can be assessed alongside your age to predict the chance of your baby suffering from Down's syndrome. If the chances seem high, amniocentesis will be offered. The triple test is not offered in all centers, although you can request it, and you may have to pay for it.

ULTRASOUND

This works by giving a photographic picture that is formed by creating images from the echoes of sound waves bouncing off different parts of the body of different consistencies. Unlike X-rays, ultrasound can show soft tissue in detail and will give a very accurate picture of the fetus in the uterus. Ultrasound is very useful as a way of determining the age of the fetus, the position of the placenta and therefore your expected date of delivery. Any visible abnormalities will be picked up clearly by the scan technician.

The first scan is often given at around 11–13 weeks of pregnancy, to establish the age of the fetus, and for nuchal translucency (see p. 79). A second scan given at 20–22 weeks will check that your baby is growing properly. The scan generally takes about 5–10 minutes.

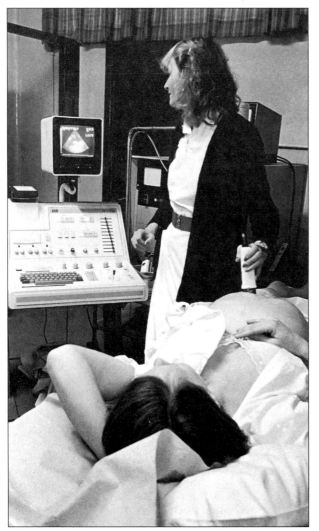

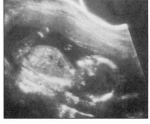

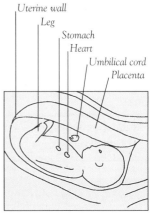

Uterine wall
Leg
Stomach
Heart
Umbilical cord
Placenta

THE FETUS IN UTERO

It is very exciting to see a picture of your baby moving about in your womb. The shapes may not make much sense to you so ask the technician to point out the head, limbs and the baby's organs. The ultrasound procedure is painless but if you have a scan in the early part of your pregnancy you will need to have a full bladder. Don't worry about this; arrive early and drink several glasses of water.

You will have been asked beforehand not to pass urine and, if it is an early scan, to drink plenty of fluids so that your bladder is full and clearly visible to the technician. Wear loose clothes so you can easily lift them off your abdomen. Warm oil or jelly is spread onto your stomach and a transducer is passed over it, which sends back signals onto a black-and-white monitor. You will feel no pain at all, just a soft, oily, flowing sensation.

USES OF ULTRASOUND

An ultrasound scan is used by medical staff to:
● help determine the age of the fetus by taking measurements of the head and body. If the scan is done early in pregnancy, it will be accurate to within one week
● measure growth, and growth retardation when clinical examination suggests something is wrong. Serial assessment—that is, a number of scans over a period of time—monitors fetal growth and establishes the estimated date of delivery
● find out the exact position of the baby and placenta before an amniocentesis (see p. 80)
● locate the position of the placenta and its condition, should it become dislodged late in pregnancy
● determine if you are carrying more than one baby should alpha-fetoprotein levels start to rise
● pick up visible abnormalities of the baby such as brain or kidney conditions
● identify any growths in the mother that might hinder delivery.

NUCHAL TRANSLUCENCY SCAN

A special scan is used to assess the risk of Down's syndrome and neural tube defects such as spina bifida and hydrocephalus. A high-definition ultrasound scan measures the fluid collected behind the baby's neck. A space of more than 2.5 mm may indicate a high risk, when considered alongside the age of the mother and her obstetric history. The test is done between weeks 11 and 13 of pregnancy, and it is about 80 percent accurate.

If your result shows the possibility of an abnormality, you may request further tests. If it shows an increased risk of spina bifida, a detailed scan of the baby's spine can check for abnormalities. If the test shows a possible risk of Down's syndrome, you will be offered an amniocentesis or CVS.

CHORIONIC VILLUS SAMPLING

This test, often shortened to CVS, is carried out at weeks 10–12 to diagnose fetal abnormalities or to assess whether the baby is at risk from certain inherited diseases, such as sickle cell anemia, hemophilia, cystic fibrosis and some metabolic errors that may lead to severe physical and mental disability. It is not a test for spina bifida, but is 100 percent accurate in detecting Down's syndrome.

The test takes about 10–20 minutes. A small sample of the chorion (the outer tissue that surrounds the developing fetus and placenta) is taken and analyzed. Using an ultrasound scan to guide the probe, a fine hollow tube is inserted in the vagina or through the abdominal wall and into the uterus. A few of the chorionic cells are sucked out; these cells are identical to those in the fetus. The chromosomal analysis of the cells taken from the chorion gives a "window" onto the fetus.

Very occasionally, CVS may lead to rupture of the amniotic sac, infection and bleeding. Even so, it only seems to increase the risk of miscarriage by one percent.

This test is performed earlier in pregnancy than amniocentesis and the results are available in about 10 days. CVS therefore gives the woman the choice of an early termination, rather than having to wait 15–18 weeks for an amniocentesis and then waiting a further three weeks for the results. If you think the test might be helpful, discuss it with your doctor or midwife early in pregnancy, as well as with your partner or a friend.

AMNIOCENTESIS

Used to detect a range of chromosomal defects, amniocentesis is not a routine test and is carried out only if certain hereditary or sex-linked disorders run in your family, or if the obstetrician suspects some abnormality that cannot be detected by other tests. Though it is readily available, it is still a serious interference with your pregnancy. It involves taking a sample of the fluid surrounding the baby in the uterus. Any discarded cells floating in the amniotic fluid will give an accurate chromosome count and denote abnormal chromosomal structure. It is also possible to find out how much oxygen and carbon dioxide is in the fluid, revealing whether the baby is getting sufficient oxygen.

Many women over 35 are concerned to see if their baby has any abnormalities. If you are worried, talk to your obstetrician. Most obstetricians will agree to this test to give you peace of mind. They will also recommend amniocentesis if you already have an abnormal child, or if there is a family history of abnormality. The sex of the baby can be determined by simply looking at some cells of the skin so you can find out if any gender-linked disorders might have been inherited. However, doctors will not do the test simply to find out the baby's sex. In cases of Rhesus incompatibility, the bilirubin content of the fluid is a good indicator as to whether the baby needs an intrauterine blood transfusion (see p. 163).

HOW AMNIOCENTESIS WORKS

Amniotic fluid is swallowed by the fetus and passed out through its mouth or bladder; this fluid contains cells from the skin and other organs that provide clues under analysis to the baby's condition. Amniocentesis is the procedure to extract this fluid from the womb. About 75 different genetic diseases can then be subjected to chromosome analysis. The test is done in a hospital or a doctor's office, generally not until 14–16 weeks after the last menstrual period; before then there is unlikely to be sufficient fluid in the amniotic sac and therefore not enough cells to analyze.

HAVING AN AMNIOCENTESIS
Amniotic fluid is drawn from the womb and then analyzed to determine the health of the baby.

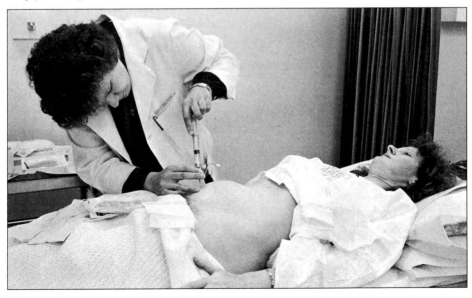

RISKS OF AMNIOCENTESIS

With a skilled operator and the use of an ultrasonic scan to show the exact position of the placenta and the fetus, the risk of miscarriage is less than that with CVS (see p. 79)—below one percent in Britain, 0.5 percent in the United States. When deciding to have amniocentesis you need to weigh up the reasons for your being offered it against the risk of miscarriage, and think about whether you are prepared to have your pregnancy terminated if the results give cause for concern.

Possibly the worst element of amniocentesis is the stress of waiting for the results, although this should be no more than three weeks. Also your amniotic fluid may only be tested for a single abnormality, which means that a negative result may not reflect other possible problems. Ask your doctor for the results of all possible tests that could apply to you.

HOW THE FLUID IS EXTRACTED

After an ultrasonic scan to determine the position of the fetus and the placenta, a small area of the abdomen is numbed with local anesthetic and a long hollow needle surmounted by a syringe is carefully inserted into the womb. About ½ oz (14 g) of fluid is then drawn out. The cells shed by the baby are then separated from the amniotic liquid in a centrifuge.

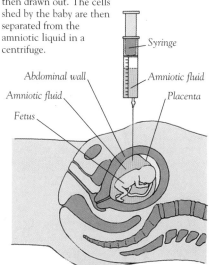

Syringe

Abdominal wall

Amniotic fluid

Amniotic fluid

Placenta

Fetus

REASONS FOR AMNIOCENTESIS

Amniocentesis will be offered if:
- you are over 35, when the risk of chromosomal abnormalities increases greatly and you may be at risk of carrying a Down's syndrome baby, for example (see below)
- you are a carrier of genetically linked disorders such as hemophilia, cystic fibrosis or certain forms of muscular dystrophy, where a male child will have a 50 percent chance of being affected
- an early cesarean section is planned. Tests on the fetal cells in the amniotic fluid can reveal the maturity of the baby's lungs so that the delivery can be timed correctly. Immature lungs may be affected by respiratory distress syndrome.

DOWN'S SYNDROME

This is the result of a chromosomal abnormality in the baby. In most cases an extra chromosome occurring before or immediately after fertilization gives the fetus 47 chromosomes in each cell instead of the normal 46 (see p. 40). The exact cause is unknown but maternal age is an important factor, the risk of having a Down's syndrome baby rising sharply after the age of 35.

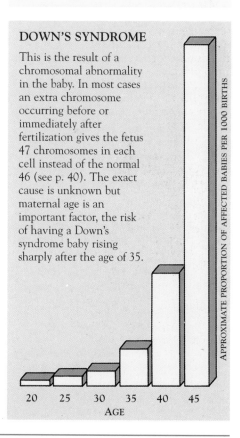

APPROXIMATE PROPORTION OF AFFECTED BABIES PER 1000 BIRTHS

20 25 30 35 40 45

AGE

81

5

The growing baby

Pregnancy can be roughly divided into three parts, or trimesters, of around 12 weeks each. By the end of the first trimester, the fetus is recognizably human despite being only 3 in. (7.5 cm) long. The second trimester is a period of rapid growth, and during the third trimester the baby gets longer and starts to accumulate fat.

Life support systems

THE MOST CRUCIAL FACTOR in the successful growth and development of your baby is a healthy placenta which forms the vital link between your body and your baby's. The placenta is the organ that allows your baby to lean on you and your body functions for its health and well-being. It also acts as a waste disposal unit and cleanses the baby's body of unwanted waste materials. It does so through its unique structure which allows the intermingling of your blood with your baby's blood. It's useful to think of the mature placenta as a blood-filled space, which is bounded on each side by a maternal surface and a fetal surface.

WHAT THE PLACENTA DOES
- Allows oxygen, nutrients and protective antibodies to be passed from mother to baby
- produces essential pregnancy hormones
- passes the baby's waste to the mother.

WHAT AMNIOTIC FLUID DOES
- Supports the fetus while it moves freely thus helping it to exercise its muscles
- maintains a constant temperature
- cushions the baby in the uterus
- exerts a constant outward pressure on the uterus so the baby has room to grow
- protects the baby's head during labor while assisting cervical dilatation
- receives substances excreted by the fetus in its urine.

AMNIOTIC FLUID

From week 4 or 5, amniotic fluid fills the amniotic space which is formed by the bag of membranes enclosing the developing embryo. By week 12 the fetus is swallowing the fluid, which is absorbed through its intestines into its bloodstream. From there it passes through the umbilical cord and the placenta and into the mother's bloodstream (see opposite). Early in the second trimester the fetus begins to use its own kidneys and to urinate.

THE MEMBRANES

These are two thin, papery sheets, the amnion and the chorion, which line the uterus and form the bag of waters inside which the baby develops.

BABY'S LIFE SUPPORT SYSTEM

The amniotic space and the placenta make up the baby's life support system. The amniotic space has developed deep inside the blastocyst, which was formed by the fertilized ovum. It therefore contains traces of cells which bear the sex of the embryo and the blueprint of its genetic makeup (see p. 40). The space is surrounded by the membranes and it contains the amniotic fluid or "liquor." The placenta is joined to the baby by the umbilical cord. This cord is made up of three intertwined blood vessels. Two carry blood from the baby to the placenta for cleansing and purification. One carries oxygenated blood and nutrients to the baby. The cord is surrounded first by a jellylike substance (Wharton's jelly) then by a membrane. The placenta itself is firmly rooted to the wall of the uterus.

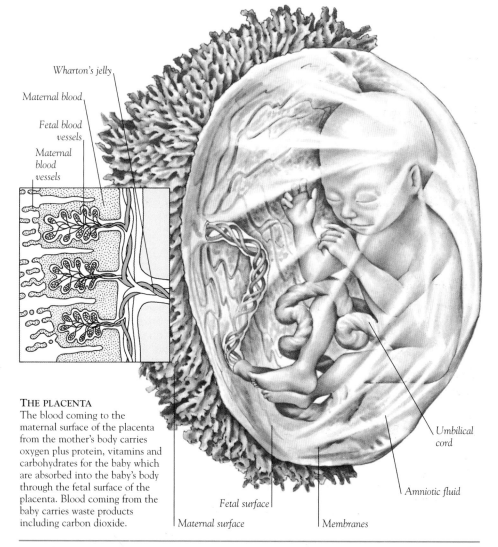

Wharton's jelly

Maternal blood

Fetal blood vessels

Maternal blood vessels

THE PLACENTA
The blood coming to the maternal surface of the placenta from the mother's body carries oxygen plus protein, vitamins and carbohydrates for the baby which are absorbed into the baby's body through the fetal surface of the placenta. Blood coming from the baby carries waste products including carbon dioxide.

Fetal surface

Maternal surface

Membranes

Umbilical cord

Amniotic fluid

First trimester

BY THE END OF THE FIRST TRIMESTER, the systems of the fetus's body are already well developed, with many organs more or less complete. Nerves and muscles are working, and reflexes are becoming established. The heart pumps about 30 liters (52 pints) of blood through its circulatory system each day. Your baby can move spontaneously, although you are not aware of these movements.

THE DEVELOPMENT OF THE EMBRYO

Between weeks 5 and 7, the embryo develops physically at a rapid rate, though it is still very small. By week 7 the intestines are formed and the limb buds are visible. The embryo is starting to look recognizably human. The small silhouettes represent the approximate size of the embryos.

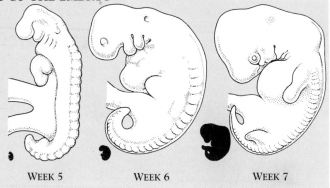

WEEK 5   **WEEK 6**   **WEEK 7**

WEEK 5

The embryo is quite easy to see with the naked eye. The spinal column is beginning to develop. The foundations of the brain and the spinal cord are appearing.
Length: 1/8 in. (2 mm)

WEEK 6

The head begins to form, followed by the chest and abdomen. The immature heart is beating. Blood cells are circulating. Blood vessels are forming in the umbilical cord to the placenta. There are small depressions where the eyes will develop and the beginnings of a mouth. The lower jaw is visible. There are arm and leg buds.
Length: 1/4 in. (6 mm)

WEEK 7

Indentations that will form the fingers and toes are visible. The intestines are almost completely formed. The lungs are formed but they are still solid. The inner parts of the ears and the eyes are developing. There are holes for the nostrils. Bone cells appear in what has thus far been cartilage bone. This marks the change from embryo to fetus.
Length: 3/4 in. (15 mm)

WEEK 8

All the internal organs are in place. The major joints of the shoulders, elbows, hips and knees are obvious. The spine can move. The genital organs are visible.
Length: 1 in. (25 mm)

WEEK 9

The mouth begins to develop and the nose is formed. The limbs, hands and feet grow rapidly. Hearing has developed. Although you are unable to feel it, your baby is moving around quite a lot.
Length: 1 1/16 in. (3 cm)
Weight: 1/16 oz (2 g)

WEEK 10

The external parts of the ears are beginning to grow and the eyes are well formed. The head is still large compared to the rest of the body and its development is pronounced. The fingers and toes are distinguishable but joined by webs of skin.
Length: 1 3/4 in. (4.5 cm)
Weight: 1/8 oz (5 g)

WEEK 11

The ovaries and testicles are formed, as are the external genital organs. The heart pumps blood to all parts of the body. By the end of week 11 all the internal organs are fully formed and functioning. Only in rare cases now will these organs be harmed by infections, chemicals or drugs.
Length: 2 3/16 in. (5.5 cm)
Weight: 5/16 oz (10 g)

WEEK 12

Closed eyelids are distinguishable as the face becomes properly formed. Muscles are starting to grow on the body which makes the limb movements more pronounced. Brain and muscles coordinate. Joints contract, toes will curl and the baby can suck. The fingers and toes are fully formed and have nails. The baby can swallow and takes in the amniotic fluid.
Length: 3 in. (7.5 cm)
Weight: 5/8 oz (18 g)

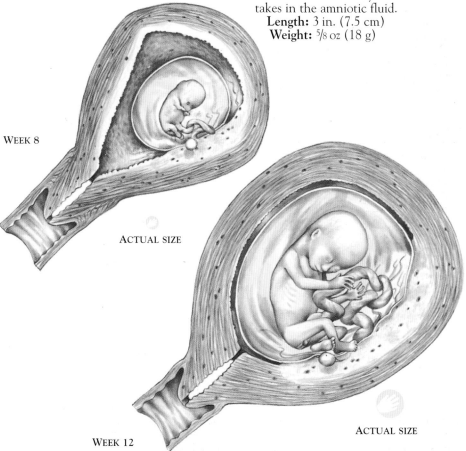

WEEK 8

ACTUAL SIZE

WEEK 12

ACTUAL SIZE

Second trimester

THE MIDDLE THIRD of pregnancy is the period in which you will feel the first fetal movements, from about week 18 onwards. Your baby is also starting to look like a real person, with hair, even eyelashes, and to behave like one when it starts to suck its thumb. After week 24 the baby is considered legally viable, that is, it is capable of sustaining independent life with special care.

WEEK 13

Your baby is completely formed. During the rest of the pregnancy it mainly grows to size, so that by the time it is born its vital organs have matured to make it capable of independent life.
Length: 3 1/2 in. (8.5 cm)
Weight: 1 oz (28 g)

WEEK 14

The increase in weight is pronounced. Major muscles respond to brain stimulation. The arms can bend from the wrist and elbow; the fingers can curl and make fists. The heart is heard with a Doppler.
Length: 4 in. (10.5 cm)
Weight: 2 1/4 oz (65 g)

WEEK 16

Limbs and joints are fully formed. Movement is vigorous, though rarely felt yet. Fine hair (lanugo) grows all over the body; eyebrows and eyelashes start to grow.
Length: 6 in. (16 cm)
Weight: 4 3/4 oz (135 g)

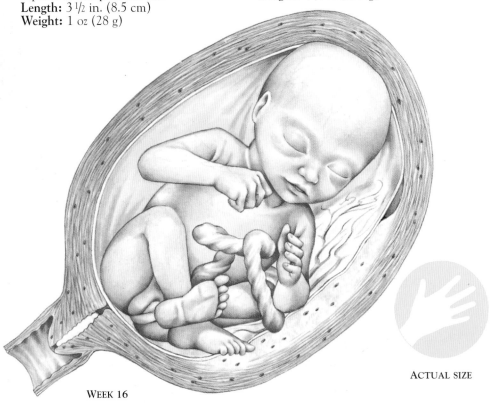

ACTUAL SIZE

WEEK 16

WEEK 20

Your baby is growing very fast. The teeth are forming in the jawbone and hair is growing on the head. The muscles are increasing in strength. Movements are more vigorous and you should feel them by now. They are light flutters rather like bubbles bursting against your abdomen.
Length: 10 in. (25 cm)
Weight: 12 oz (340 g)

WEEK 24

The baby intermittently sucks its thumb and it can cough and hiccup. It hasn't yet laid down fat stores and is still thin.
Length: 13 in. (33 cm)
Weight: 1¼ lb (570 g)

WEEK 28

The head is now more in proportion to the body. Fat stores are beginning to accumulate. The body is covered in thick grease (vernix) which prevents the skin from becoming soggy from immersion in the amniotic fluid. The lungs are reaching maturity and the baby has a good chance of survival—about 80 percent—if born.
Length: 14½ in. (37 cm)
Weight: 2 lb (900 g)

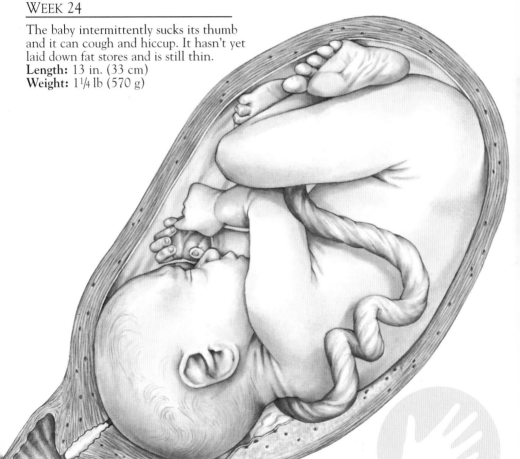

WEEK 28   ACTUAL SIZE

Third trimester

IF BORN DURING the third trimester before the 38th week, the baby might have breathing problems and difficulty keeping itself warm. However, with modern special care facilities the baby has a good chance of survival—about 80 percent at 28 weeks, and rising the closer to term (40 weeks) that it is born.

WEEK 32

Your baby's proportions are as you would expect them to be at birth. It is much stronger and in over 90 percent of cases it lies with its head down towards your pelvis. Its movements are now very vigorous and clearly discernible.
Length: 16 in. (40.5 cm)
Weight: 3 1/2 lb (1.6 kg)

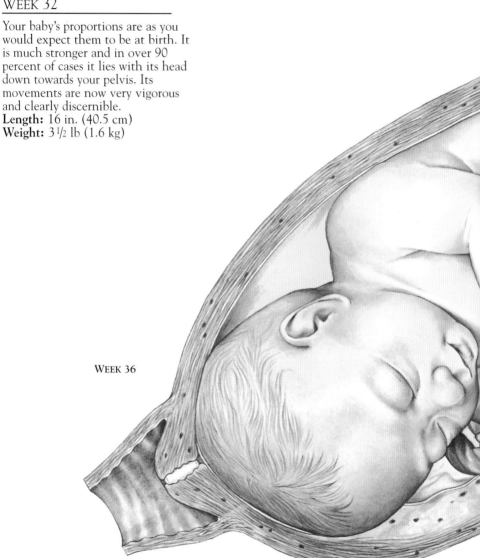

WEEK 36

WEEK 36

During the next four weeks the baby gains about 1 oz (28 g) a day. It fills the uterus and the movements are no less frequent, but are more like jabs as its space is restricted and it settles into the position for birth. The irises of the eyes are blue.

The soft nails have grown to the end of the toes and fingers. Hair on the head can be up to 1–2 in. (2.5–5 cm) long. In a boy the testes should have descended. If this is a first baby the head will usually descend into the pelvis by now.
Length: 18 in. (46 cm)
Weight: 5 1/2 lb (2.5 kg)

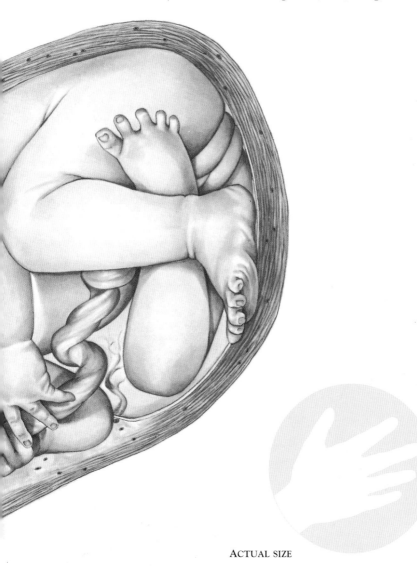

ACTUAL SIZE

Full term

FORTY WEEKS AFTER the first day of your last menstrual period your baby is ready to be born, though babies rarely arrive on the estimated day of delivery (see p. 49).

With second and subsequent babies, the head engages in the bony pelvic opening about one week before the birth or in some cases not until labor has started.

WEEK 40

The vernix has decreased so that there are only remnants in the skin folds—around the neck, armpits and groin. The nails on the fingers are long and will need cutting shortly after birth. When the baby is awake its eyes are open and it can discern light. Most of the lanugo has gone.
Length: 20 in. (51 cm)
Weight: 7 1/2 lb (3.4 kg)

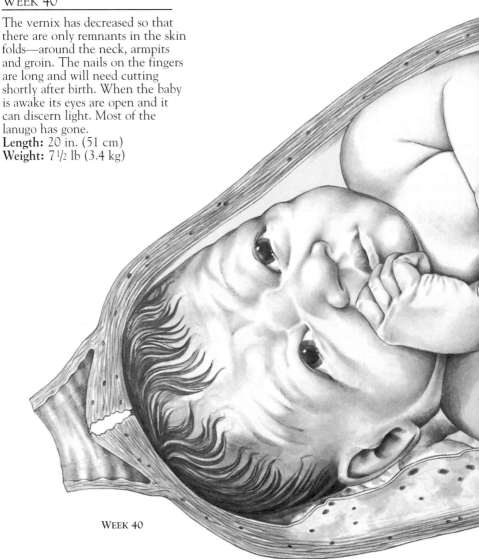

WEEK 40

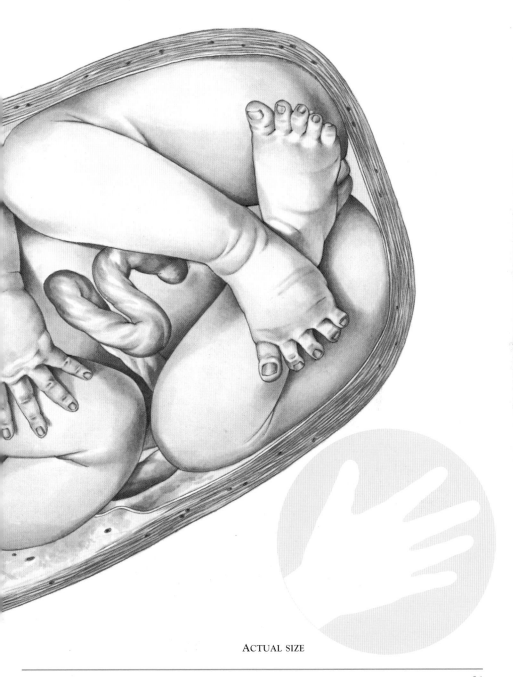

ACTUAL SIZE

6

Physical changes

Nearly all the changes in your body that you can see and feel, such as enlargement of the breasts, deepening pigmentation of the skin, and slight breathlessness on exertion, are due in one way or another to the increased production of a range of pregnancy hormones. Early in pregnancy your ovaries are responsible for the main output, but very quickly the maternal supply begins to be overtaken by that from the placenta. The output of hormones is colossal. For instance, during the menstrual cycle, the maximum daily output of one key hormone, progesterone, would be a few milligrams a day, but towards the end of pregnancy this rises to as much as 250 mg a day. While progesterone output increases 50–60 times, that of another key hormone, estrogen, increases 20–30 times. These hormones cause changes in your whole body's structure and processes so that it can support and nourish your developing baby throughout pregnancy.

The menstrual cycle

THE FIRST DEVIATION from normal hormonal patterns occurs very early in pregnancy. The menstrual cycle begins when a hormone (follicle-stimulating hormone—FSH) from the pituitary gland stimulates the development of an egg (ovum) in a follicle inside one of the ovaries (see p. 42). In a 28-day menstrual cycle (see p. 39), ovulation occurs around day 14 when the follicle bursts, discharging the ovum which starts to move down the fallopian tube towards the uterus. It is helped by "fingers" at the end of the fallopian tube which direct it on its way. At the same time, the lining of the uterus (endometrium) begins to

thicken and the mucus at the neck of the uterus (cervix) becomes thinner so that the sperm can gain an easier entry. If the ovum is not fertilized, at around day 24 the decaying follicle (corpus luteum) begins to wither, and further hormonal changes result in shedding of the endometrium and bleeding on day 28 and day 1 of the next cycle.

When pregnancy occurs, fertilization happens around day 14 of the cycle, then implantation of the fertilized ovum in the uterine wall begins some seven days after that, around day 21. There are three or four days between implantation and the usual regression of the corpus luteum. The body has only this short interval in which to stop the regression and suppress menstruation. This is probably achieved by a powerful hormone called human chorionic gonadotrophin (HCG), which is produced by the fertilized ovum and whose immediate function is thought to be the maintenance of a healthy corpus luteum and the levels of estrogen and progesterone coming from the ovaries. In this way, the mother's body and the developing embryo, which at this stage is only a minute ball of cells (see p. 42), cooperate to keep the pregnancy intact.

The hormone levels of some pregnant women are not sufficiently increased to prevent some bleeding at the time of their first missed period. Slight breakthrough bleeding may occur at the time when the second and even third missed periods would have been due. The bleeding does not harm the baby. However, if hormonal levels are too low, a miscarriage will almost certainly occur (see p. 160).

THE PLACENTA

At implantation, part of the fertilized ovum puts out microscopic protrusions (chorionic villi) which embed themselves in the uterine wall. These villi become the placenta, which supplies food and oxygen to the baby and carries waste from it. During the first trimester, the placenta develops into an efficient chemical factory, producing an ever-increasing supply of pregnancy hormones that alter the mother's body to maintain the pregnancy and prepare for lactation, and also maintain healthy reproductive organs and the efficient function of the placenta, so keeping the baby well nourished.

28-DAY MENSTRUAL CYCLE

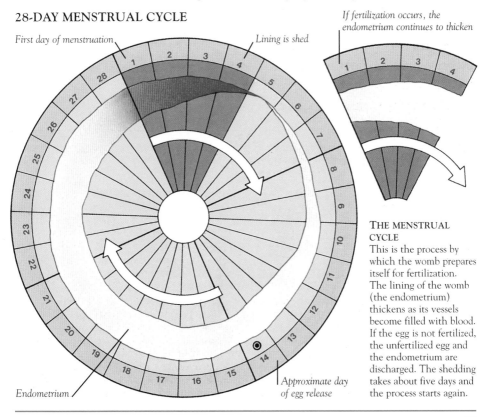

First day of menstruation

Lining is shed

If fertilization occurs, the endometrium continues to thicken

Endometrium

Approximate day of egg release

THE MENSTRUAL CYCLE
This is the process by which the womb prepares itself for fertilization. The lining of the womb (the endometrium) thickens as its vessels become filled with blood. If the egg is not fertilized, the unfertilized egg and the endometrium are discharged. The shedding takes about five days and the process starts again.

HORMONES OF PREGNANCY

NAME	ACTION	EFFECT ON MOTHER & BABY
HUMAN CHORIONIC GONADOTROPHIN (HCG)	Produced by the chorionic villi. Causes the ovary to produce more progesterone (see below), thus suppressing menstruation and sustaining the pregnancy. Reaches a peak of production around the 70th day and then falls to a constant value for the rest of the pregnancy. Maintains the function of the ovaries until the placenta takes over.	High levels in the bloodstream parallel the time when women normally suffer from nausea in pregnancy (see p. 47). Could be associated with morning sickness. Detection of this hormone in urine is a reliable pregnancy test (see p. 48).
HUMAN PLACENTAL LACTOGEN (HPL)	Produced by the placenta, it is essential to normal milk production.	Enlarges the breasts and causes secretion of colostrum from about the fifth month.
RELAXIN	Probably produced by the placenta. In animal experiments, it was found to soften the uterine cervix. Relaxes the pelvic joints.	May have an effect of relaxing the ligaments and joints.
ESTROGEN	Produced in the placenta using starter substances from the mother's and the baby's adrenal glands.	Affects all aspects of pregnancy. It is particularly important in maintaining the health of the genital tract, the reproductive organs and the breasts.
PROGESTERONE	Produced in the same way as estrogen. Sustains the pregnancy, relaxes smooth muscle.	Affects all aspects of pregnancy. Prepares the breasts for lactation. Relaxation of joints and ligaments in preparation for childbirth can affect bowel movements, causing constipation, and can result in back pain (see p. 148). Raises body temperature.
MELANOCYTE STIMULATING HORMONE (MSH)	Produced in higher levels than normal during pregnancy. Stimulates the skin to produce pigment.	Increase in color of the nipples, patches of brown pigmentation on the face, inner thighs and a brown line running down the center of the abdomen (see p. 100). Some women notice none of these changes.

Breasts

SIZE AND SHAPE VARY from individual to individual and according to the point in the menstrual cycle. In the second half of the cycle, after ovulation day, most women experience some enlargement of their breasts. Just before menstruation, the consistency becomes rather nodular as the milk glands enlarge, the tinted areas around the nipples (areolas) become slightly bumpy as the sebaceous glands enlarge, and the nipples become sensitive.

Changes in the breasts may be one of the earliest signs of pregnancy that you become aware of. Most women with an average 28-day cycle will notice a definite enlargement of the breasts by week 6–8 of

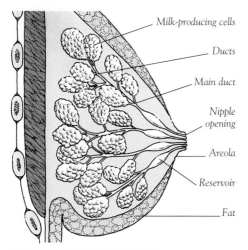

Milk-producing cells

Ducts

Main duct

Nipple opening

Areola

Reservoir

Fat

CROSS-SECTION OF THE BREAST
The breast is prepared for lactation during pregnancy by the action of estrogen and progesterone.

pregnancy, two to four weeks after their first missed period would have started. The breasts will feel firm and generally tender and have more and larger veins than usual running close to the surface of the skin. Tingling is common, as are occasional stabbing pains. The sebaceous glands on the areolas (Montgomery's tubercles) become raised, nodular and pink.

The breasts are composed mainly of millions of tiny milk glands, plus their small ducts, that join to come out at the nipple. Although there is almost certainly some overlap in the effect of hormones, estrogen stimulates the growth of the ducts while progesterone stimulates enlargement of the glands themselves. From early pregnancy your breasts will be making a form of milk called colostrum (see p. 221). This may be secreted involuntarily; it's nothing to worry about.

Most of the growth of the ducts and increase in size and weight of the breasts occurs in the first trimester. It is at this point that you should be fitted for a good bra. You will probably need one at least two sizes larger. You will also need feeding bras after the baby is born (see p. 137). These should be fitted around a month before the baby is due. If you support the weight of your breasts during pregnancy and lactation they should return to their prepregnant shape and firmness when you stop breastfeeding. Some women find their breasts are smaller after weaning as the original fat in the breasts has been replaced by milk-producing ducts. Towards the end of the first trimester you will see one of the last changes in the breasts, darkening of the nipples and areolas due to a general increase in pigmentation (see p. 100) which is another characteristic of pregnancy.

INVERTED NIPPLES

If your nipples do not protrude when you are cold, sexually excited or breastfeeding, they are said to be flat or inverted. Your breasts will be examined during your first examination at the prenatal clinic and any inversion noted. You can improve inverted nipples by wearing breast shields under your bra or you can try an exercise known as the Hoffmann technique. Place an index finger either side of the areola and stretch the nipples. Repeat this with your fingers placed above and below the areola. Do this a couple of times a day during pregnancy. The baby may help to solve the problem but could have difficulty latching on.

FLAT OR INVERTED NIPPLES
You can improve them by wearing breast shields under your bra from about week 15. Wear them for a few hours at first, building up to several hours each day in the third trimester. Made of plastic or glass, they have a hole in them through which the nipple is gently pulled by suction. It is not painful.

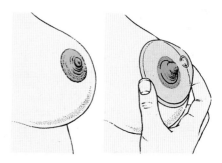

The uterus

THREE PRINCIPAL TASKS are performed by the uterus during pregnancy. It is the site of implantation by the fertilized ovum, it accommodates the growing baby, and it expels the baby at term. To achieve the second of these tasks the uterus has to grow and distend, while restraining a normal tendency to contract when there is something inside it and while the outlet, the cervix, remains resistant to stretching.

EXPANSION

To accommodate the developing baby, placenta and surrounding fluids, the internal volume of the uterus has to expand from being a potential space to one of about 9 pints (5 liters)—an increase in volume of some 1000 times. In the first half of pregnancy, the uterus gains weight quickly, mainly due to an increase in the size of the muscle fibers. Each muscle cell of the uterus increases in size by as much as 50 times, initially under the stimulation of estrogen. Around midpregnancy this rate of growth slows down, but uterine volume then increases rapidly. The uterus increases its weight some 20 times, from about 1½ oz (40 g) to 28 oz (800 g) at term. The expansion is not noticeable until about week 16 when the uterus begins to rise out of the pelvis. By week 36 the top of the uterus has risen to just below the breast bone. When the baby's head engages (see p. 171), it descends again.

THE EXPANDING UTERUS
The uterus increases its volume about 1000 times in pregnancy and as it does, it crowds out the other organs. This can result in problems such as frequent urination, heartburn, breathlessness and constipation.

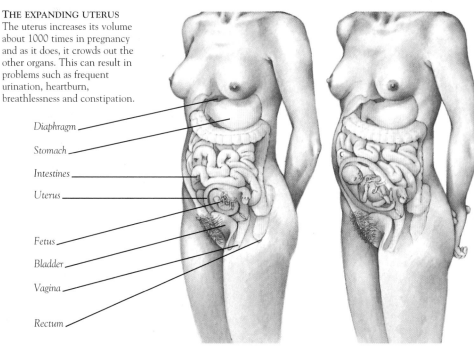

Diaphragm

Stomach

Intestines

Uterus

Fetus

Bladder

Vagina

Rectum

12 WEEKS
The uterus can just be felt by abdominal palpitation as it emerges out of the pelvic cavity.

16 WEEKS
The uterus is expanding quickly, your waist disappears and you are noticeably pregnant.

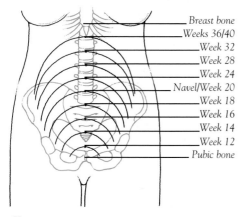

Breast bone
Weeks 36/40
Week 32
Week 28
Week 24
Navel/Week 20
Week 18
Week 16
Week 14
Week 12
Pubic bone

THE HEIGHT OF THE FUNDUS
This can be determined by abdominal palpitation (feeling the abdomen) or by measuring from the pubic bone. It is sometimes used as a guide to the duration of your pregnancy and is written on your notes.

CONTRACTIONS

One of the normal characteristics of uterine muscle is that it undergoes contractions which are hardly ever felt. All the way through pregnancy the uterus contracts in a weak, short-lived way that you may or may not notice, although if you put a hand on your abdomen you can feel the muscle going tight and hard. These slight, painless movements are called Braxton Hicks contractions and occur about every 20 minutes throughout pregnancy. They are important as they ensure a good blood circulation through the uterus and they help uterine growth. You probably won't notice Braxton Hicks contractions until the last month of your pregnancy. They can become quite strong and may be mistaken for labor. This is called "false labor" (see p. 173).

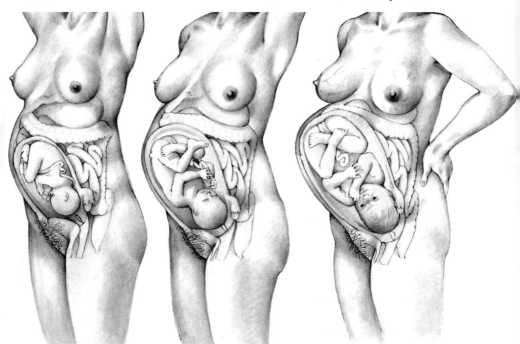

28 WEEKS
The skin on your stomach will start to stretch and the upward pressure may lead to indigestion.

36 WEEKS
The uterus is now putting pressure on your ribcage and you may feel a jabbing pain there.

40 WEEKS
The baby's head will engage in the pelvic cavity and put pressure on the groin and the pelvis.

Up until weeks 12–14, the developing baby can quite easily be accommodated in the space within the growing uterus, but after this time the junction of the uterus and the top of the cervix begins to smooth out, giving the baby more space. This part is called the lower segment of the uterus. While the upper half of the cervix is muscular and stretchy, the lower half contains a strong, tight band of fibrous tissue. This helps to prevent the cervix from dilating before the baby is ready to be born.

Although this band of fibrous tissue softens during the last weeks of pregnancy to prepare for the birth, its resistance to dilatation is usually sufficient to withstand Braxton Hicks contractions. During labor, it is the upper segment of the uterus that contracts to push the baby out.

Vagina

EARLY IN PREGNANCY, the vaginal tissues also change so that the vagina will dilate more easily for the birth. The muscle cells enlarge and the mucous membranes of the lining thicken. One side effect of this is an increase in vaginal secretions (see p. 154) which may mean you need light sanitary pads for comfort.

If the secretion has an offensive smell or makes you sore, tell your doctor and never douche during pregnancy. One other result of this increased lubrication and swelling of the vagina may be an increase in sexual pleasure. This, however, differs from woman to woman and will vary throughout the pregnancy (see p. 106).

Vital functions

YOUR BODY WILL REACT to the hormonal stimulation of pregnancy with widespread changes in the important circulatory, respiratory and urinary systems. It used to be thought that the relationship between the mother and embryo was simply that of host and parasite but we now know that it is much more complex. From the earliest days, in response to the diversified and raised hormonal output, the mother continually anticipates the needs of her baby: by changes in her vital functions, she precedes the baby's demands.

BLOOD

An average-sized, nonpregnant woman has about 9 pints (5 liters) of circulating blood. During pregnancy, the volume of blood increases by about 2½ pints (1.5 liters). The volume gradually increases from about week 10, reaching a plateau in the third trimester. The extra blood is required by the uterus (which takes about 25 percent), the breasts and other vital organs—even the gums receive an increase in their blood supply (see p. 101). The increase in the liquid part of the blood (plasma) is proportionately greater than that of the red cells. If the red cells become too diluted, this will show up in prenatal blood tests as a fall in the hemoglobin concentration and this is known as physiological anemia. It is not the same thing as iron-deficiency anemia (see p. 156). In a normal pregnant woman, the number of red blood cells multiplies steadily, particularly if you include a lot of iron in your diet.

Another effect of the increase of fluids circulating in the body is a lowering of the sodium concentration, which is why you shouldn't restrict your salt intake during pregnancy (see p. 115) unless you have serious fluid retention.

HEART

With more fluids to push around the body, the heart has extra work to do. By the end of the second trimester it has increased its workload by 40 percent. It enlarges to accommodate this extra work but astonishingly your pulse rate is hardly raised from its prepregnant level. Much of the circulation increase is directed to the uterus. Blood flow to the kidneys also increases as does the blood flowing through your skin, so that it is warmer and sweats more. During the third trimester, the uterus may press on the large vein in the abdomen if you lie on your back. This causes blood pressure to fall and may make you feel dizzy and faint.

LUNGS

To keep blood well supplied with oxygen, the lungs have to work harder. Take plenty of fresh air and exercise, so that the blood supply to the lungs will be improved. During the third trimester, the uterus will begin to crowd the lungs out. You may feel uncomfortable, and find yourself having to take deep breaths. Sitting up straight helps, even in bed.

KIDNEYS

Your kidneys have to filter and clean 50 percent more blood than they did before. As a result, all renal function becomes more efficient, the body getting rid of waste products like urea and uric acid faster than before. But the kidneys don't distinguish between waste products and nutrients, so glucose is also quickly cleared from the blood, together with minerals and vitamins—for instance, water-soluble vitamin C, plus folic acid which is excreted at four or five times the usual rate. This is one of the reasons for making sure your vitamin and mineral intake is maintained during pregnancy, and why you may need folic acid supplements (see pp. 35 and 114). In addition to the greater amount of urine to be got rid of, you will probably find you need to pass urine more frequently than usual as the contracting uterus irritates the neighboring bladder. This is one of the earliest signs of pregnancy (see p. 47). Even though it is annoying, don't restrict your fluid intake.

JOINTS

The ligaments that surround, connect and support the joints are softened and become more flexible, especially in the pelvis, due to the action of pregnancy hormones. In labor the joints of the pelvis can stretch, allowing your baby a smooth passage to the outside world.

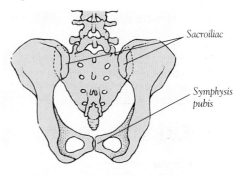

Sacroiliac

Symphysis pubis

SACROILIAC JOINT
It is located at the top of the buttocks and can be associated with low back pain.

Joints affected include the sacroiliac joint, and the junction of the pubic bones at the front, the symphysis pubis.

After about week 16, the weight of the growing baby pushing down in the pelvis can tip the pelvic brim forward. The changed angle puts strain on the muscles and ligaments surrounding the lower spine, and may cause backache. You can counter the forward tilt with good posture and by doing pelvic tilt exercises (see p. 130).

Other ligaments are also likely to stretch and ache, particularly in the legs and feet. Good posture (see p. 120), exercise, shoes with some support and massage (see p. 145) can do a lot to counteract discomfort (see pp. 148–155).

Skin

THOUGH SOME WOMEN DO GLOW with good health during pregnancy, there are some changes to the skin that are not so flattering, but they usually disappear shortly after the birth of the baby.

PIGMENTATION

Some degree of darkening is a universal characteristic of pregnancy, although its depth varies according to skin color. Blonds, redheads, and even brunettes who have pale skin may see little change, whereas olive-skinned women may find that their whole skin darkens and areas like the nipples, abdomen and genital region remain dark brown after delivery.

Pigmentation of the nipples and areolas and a dark line down the center of the abdomen, called the linea nigra, usually make their appearance around week 14. The linea nigra can be up to $1/2$ in. (1 cm) wide and stretches from the pubic hair to the navel, or even up to the breast bone. The navel tends to darken, and by the third trimester it stretches, becoming completely flat by 40 weeks. It returns to normal after delivery. The linea nigra also begins to fade shortly after delivery, but may take several months to disappear completely, or remain as a shadow.

Any brown birthmarks, moles, freckles, or recent scars, particularly on the abdomen, may darken during pregnancy. The effect becomes more obvious after exposure to sunlight, but will probably return to normal shortly after delivery. Blotchy and irregular brown patches (chloasma) sometimes appear and are made worse by sunlight (see p. 138). They usually begin to fade shortly after delivery and may disappear completely in a few months.

TEXTURE

It's impossible to anticipate whether your skin, particularly on your face, will become drier or oilier, improve or get worse during pregnancy. High levels of hormones have several effects on skin, as does the greater amount of blood circulating to it. Oiliness results from the action of progesterone, which encourages the secretion of sebum. Spots can appear unexpectedly (see p. 139) because of fluctuating hormone levels, not just on the face, but on the back too. Increased fluid retention can fill out lines or cause unwelcome puffiness (see p. 139), depending on your face shape. However, these changes are all normal and will disappear after your baby is born.

STRETCHMARKS

These occur in the skin under several different conditions. The first is in adolescence when we grow quickly. The second is whenever we put on a large amount of weight in a short time, and the third is during pregnancy. The underlying cause is always the same—tearing of collagen bundles. Collagen is the "skeleton" of the skin; its network of elastic bundles allows the skin to stretch with movement or with a change in size or shape. The marks in pregnancy are due to the high level of sex hormones that are circulating in the blood. One of the effects of these hormones is to break down and remove protein from the skin, thereby disrupting the collagen bundles and making the skin thin and papery. It appears delicate and stretchy in certain areas—the stretchmarks.

The stretchmarks that occur when we put on a lot of weight result when the collagen bundles are stretched to the point of breaking by the fat, which is laid down underneath the skin.

During pregnancy, these marks appear on the breasts, the abdomen, and also on the thighs and buttocks. They will remain pinkish throughout pregnancy, but after delivery they shrink and become a silvery color after nine months or so (see p. 152).

Hair and nails

THESE ARE BOTH MADE from the same substance—keratin—and you may or may not notice any changes to your hair (see also p. 138) and fingernails.

HAIR CHANGES

Pregnancy can have an unpredictable and quite dramatic effect on hair. Curls may straighten out or straight hair become curly, and these changes can remain after your baby is born. Some women's hair becomes luxuriant and shiny, others' lifeless or greasy. Even body hair may become more or less apparent.

Most women's hair becomes more oily, particularly towards the end of the pregnancy, due to the very high levels of progesterone in the blood, which stimulate the sebaceous glands on the scalp. Dry hair may benefit from this change, though it can make hair lank. If you've always had normal hair, you may find any change difficult to live with because your hair won't be as predictable as it was before. Because of this unpredictability, pregnancy is not a good time to dye your hair or have a perm.

One reason hair may become progressively thicker is that hormonal changes cause more than 90 percent of the hair on your head to be thrown simultaneously into a growing phase (normally only 90 percent are growing and the remainder resting). Therefore during pregnancy, your hair should be thicker and stronger, although this will not apply to every woman.

Soon after birth the hair that you would normally lose, but didn't because of your pregnancy, will be lost in large amounts, making way for the new. Hair loss can go on for anything up to 18 months and, if replacement is too slow, the hair becomes thinner and thinner. This can be alarming, but no woman has gone bald simply as a result of pregnancy, so be assured that your hair will eventually recover.

Facial and body hair goes into a growing phase, too, which may increase its quantity and strength. Women with dark skin, in whom pregnancy causes a greatly increased amount of pigmentation, may find that their body and facial hair darkens. In some cases this hair does not return to its former color.

NAIL CHANGES

Splitting and breaking of nails is another problem for some women in pregnancy. Use rubber gloves and hand lotion to protect the nails. They will return to normal after delivery, although those who have stronger, shinier nails in pregnancy may suffer brittleness after delivery.

Teeth and gums

IT USED TO BE SAID that a baby absorbed the calcium from its mother's teeth and therefore women were more susceptible to tooth decay during pregnancy than at other times. This is not so, as there is no way of extracting calcium from the teeth. However, the high levels of progesterone that are produced during pregnancy will make the margins of the gums around the teeth soft and spongy, predisposing them to infection (see p. 148). It is therefore essential that you are meticulous about oral hygiene and avoid the sugary foods that lead to tooth decay. Make an appointment to see your dentist as soon as you know you are pregnant and keep up your regular checkups throughout pregnancy and lactation. Remember to tell your dentist that you are pregnant as you should avoid X-rays.

7

Emotional changes

Psychologically speaking, your main task during pregnancy is to incorporate your new baby into your long-term planning, your future, your feelings and your lifestyle. Though these challenges are similar for men and women, you can be affected differently. Any emotional turmoil you feel is a positive force to guide you through your adjustment to becoming a mother or father, helping you to be emotionally well prepared for your new baby. The fact that you may have second thoughts doesn't mean that you've made a mistake. It would be wrong to think that having a baby is all fun. The best thing you can do is to be open about your feelings. If you talk to each other honestly, you will clarify your thinking and prepare the basis for a constant exchange throughout the pregnancy.

Self-image

THE CHANGING SIZE AND SHAPE of your body may make you feel strange about yourself, and you may even worry about becoming fat or unattractive to your partner. Try to be positive about your shape. Look for the beauty in the fullness of your breasts and the curve of your abdomen. For both men and women, a pregnant body is extremely sensuous and a pregnant woman is beautiful in her own way. Your image of yourself in this condition is important. Feeling proud of your shape and your fertility will make you more positive about your condition and encourage you to take a general interest in looking good (see p. 134), being healthy (see p. 111) and keeping fit (see pp. 120–133).

HOW HORMONES AFFECT MOOD

Mood changes are largely a reflection of the tremendous change in hormonal secretions, so there's no need to feel guilty about them. The upheaval of pregnancy makes nearly all women feel emotionally fragile, prone to crying and feelings of panic. Even in the most positive of pregnancies you may feel some confusion. Once you know it's normal to feel low, you'll feel better and your moods will pass more quickly. Try not to be too analytical; react to the next thing that comes along.

YOUR CHANGING SHAPE
You should feel confident and proud of your rounded body: think of it as a reaffirmation of life.

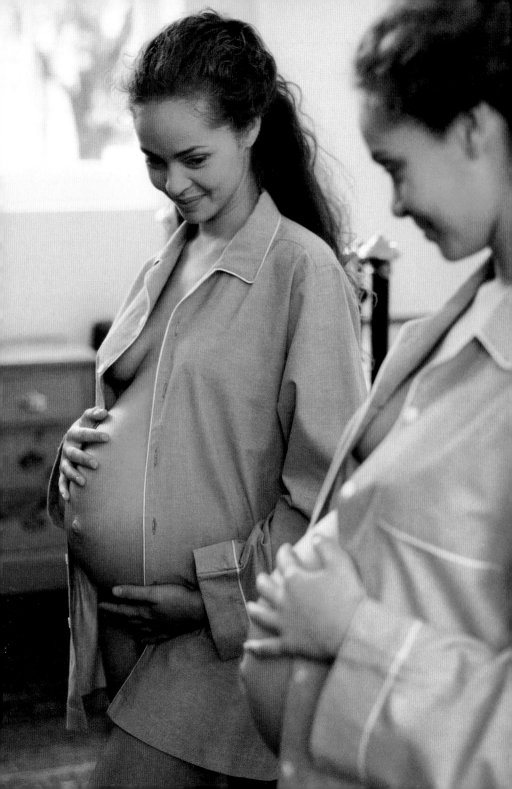

Feelings about your partner

THE CHANGE FROM BEING an individual to being a parent is one of the most profound you'll ever experience; a woman is different from a mother; a father is not the same as a man. Approaching parenthood together is an essentially positive and deeply satisfying experience but you're going to find it shattering, exhausting and incredibly hard work too.

There are going to be many ups and downs for you and your partner to cope with during pregnancy. Be prepared for them and give them time and patience.

If you're in a good partnership, one of the things that you'll almost certainly feel is that the pregnancy cements your relationship. If you can, try to go away for a weekend or have a holiday when you're between four and seven months pregnant (the time when most women feel at their best), as it will give you a chance to share your feelings and help you look forward to the exciting times ahead.

The strengthening of your bonds may be a little claustrophobic at first until you get used to it. It might help if you agree from the very beginning that you'll talk about things relating to the pregnancy in an open way, and that you won't interpret your partner's comments as rejection or unkindness. During this time it's quite common for couples to make unusual demands on each other as a test of loyalty and devotion, but try to be realistic about small grievances and be quick to point them out and explain them to each other. The reality of approaching parenthood can sometimes cause tension, but this can usually be defused if you decide to be frank with each other. Friction and conflict seem to diminish when each partner is prepared to be generous towards the other.

You'll certainly start evaluating each other in the light of your new roles. You may have always had an image of the kind of parent you would want your partner to be and you'll try to see how he or she measures up to your fantasy. Don't be too hard in your evaluation of your partner; think about how you would feel by evaluating yourself in the same way. This will make you sympathetic towards your partner's feelings about being judged all the time.

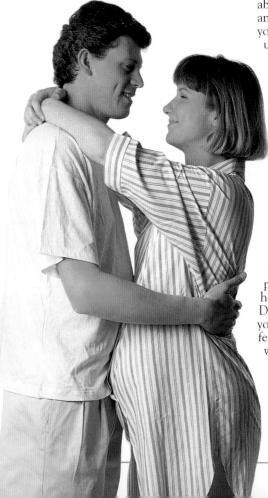

INCREASED INTIMACY
The special bond of pregnancy brings many couples much closer together and helps to deepen their relationship.

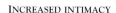

BEING AN INVOLVED FATHER

Every father needs to take an active rather than a passive role in a fundamental life event such as the birth of his child. You need to feel that you really are contributing something as well and, even better, that you're taking this important step together.

Becoming a father doesn't start with the birth of your child: it helps to get involved with your partner's pregnancy from the beginning, to understand what is going on in her body and to understand the physical and emotional pressures she is experiencing. Nearly all women are helped by the presence of their partner at the first prenatal visit, for example.

As a prospective father, you may be wondering how you can help your partner through her pregnancy while making sure that your own needs are met, but you have to be prepared for your life to be disrupted to some extent. The golden rule is to be observant of your partner's needs, to assist in her care, and to be closely linked with everything that's happening to her. Fatherhood always involves hard work, a lot of responsibility and a considerable amount of time but will repay you with immeasurable joy, satisfaction and happiness. During pregnancy, the delivery and after the birth, your partner will be depending on you for courage and support. If she doesn't get them from you she will feel alone, which is bad for her and for your baby.

It's not uncommon for a father-to-be to discover feelings of jealousy towards his partner and her condition during a first pregnancy. You may feel neglected if your partner seems more ready to share information about her pregnancy with women friends rather than with you. If you find that you are trying to minimize her requests, her problems and needs, take a look at yourself. Make a special effort to be reasonable, and listen, sympathize and encourage. She will almost certainly return your gifts, which means acceptance of you not only as lover but now also as the father of your child.

The interdependence on one another is not easy in practice and certain traditions of bringing up boys don't facilitate it. The strong, silent loner doesn't easily make an involved father. It's easier to learn from a good parent who acts as an example, but you may have to educate yourself into fatherhood by devising your own way of learning.

It may hearten you to know that mothers and fathers start off more or less equally ignorant about babies and small children. Mothers do eventually learn something out of necessity and trial and error. Unless you're involved, you'll not even be that lucky. It's a tragedy to miss out on the care of your child and instead remain a kind of stranger. Also remember that there's no one right or wrong way to be a parent, but you have to be ready to grow just as your child is growing—in caring, in admitting mistakes, and in making time available among your family members. All these things will help to make you a better father.

Special anxieties

NEARLY EVERY PROSPECTIVE parent, but particularly a mother, is beset by anxieties about the baby, especially in the last trimester. The immediacy of delivery and having a new baby nurtures natural anxieties about whether the baby will have any kind of abnormality, whether you will be a capable parent, whether you will do something silly like dropping the baby and whether you will be able to cope with the day-to-day care in the first weeks. All of these feelings are quite natural and most women harbor them. If you know that they are going to occur and are normal and natural, this will help to defuse your anxiety.

Dreams in particular can be disturbing. You may dream of mistreating your baby or not caring for it properly. You may dream of losing the baby or that it is stillborn. Your dreams represent a perfectly legitimate fear in both these respects; fear that you have at the back of your mind, but during your waking hours are not prepared to face. Think of your dreams as a release for your anxieties. The fact that you may dream about harming your baby doesn't mean that you really want to harm it or ever would; it's a healthy symptom of wanting to do the best for your baby.

Every pregnant woman at some stage worries about something being wrong with the baby. Dreaming about losing the baby or about having a stillbirth has little foundation in reality. It's more likely to do with figuratively losing the baby from your uterus. Dreams about the baby dying are part of your understandable concern for your baby's well-being. One way of dealing with them is to try to put them out of your head upon waking and get on with some pleasurable aspect of preparing for the baby's arrival.

All women worry about how they'll behave in labor. Will the pain be too much? Will they scream? Will their bowels or bladder empty embarrassingly? Will they lose control of themselves and act foolishly? Such fears are normal and the chances are you'll be surprised at how calmly you behave, though most of us do something rather silly at some time during the labor and birth. It isn't important. Remember midwives and doctors have seen it all before; you can't embarrass them.

Sex in pregnancy

THE MAJORITY OF WOMEN I have spoken to about sex and pregnancy have almost universally felt that sex was better than ever. Because of the high level of circulating hormones, a woman can become stimulated more readily and reach a high pitch of sexual excitement more quickly than in the nonpregnant state. Many parts of her body, such as the breasts, nipples and genital area (see p. 98), are more sensitive during pregnancy because all the sexual organs become highly developed and more capable of arousal than before pregnancy occurred. Also there is the freedom from having to use contraceptive methods.

There does, however, tend to be some loss of libido during the first and third trimesters. This could be a result of increased hormonal activity at the beginning of pregnancy, causing nausea and tiredness, and of your large shape at the end. Even if you don't feel like making love, and many couples don't, explore other ways of touching and giving sexual pleasure to each other.

There doesn't seem to be any medical reason why you should not enjoy full sexual intercourse throughout your pregnancy, as the womb is completely sealed off by the mucus plug. However, an article in one of Britain's medical journals entitled "Does sex embarrass the fetus?" did point out that a great deal of sexual activity might encourage maternal infections. But the report showed that this was probably related to other factors including hygiene, even possibly different sexual partners.

As long as you only have sex with your partner, and only when you feel like it, and as long as it isn't too athletic, sex is to be recommended throughout pregnancy, unless your doctor advises you otherwise or other factors relate to your condition (see opposite). Sex is good for your body too – orgasm exercises the uterine muscles, though this can cause contractions later on in pregnancy, which die down after a few minutes. Sex also helps you to become more aware of your pelvic floor muscles.

WILL SEX HARM THE BABY?

There is no information suggesting that sex harms the baby. Sex cannot introduce infection to the baby because it is safely protected in a surrounding bag of fluid. Sex will not crush the baby either. The bag of fluid (amniotic sac—see p. 83) is an excellent cushion and once the baby is firmly attached to its mother's uterus, there is no way that intercourse can cause a miscarriage. If the baby should miscarry it will be for reasons other than the fact you are having sexual intercourse, as will the onset of labor. Labor will not start simply because of the stimulation of sex.

WHEN NOT TO HAVE SEX

● If bleeding occurs, consult your doctor immediately and refrain from further intercourse. It may not be serious but your doctor has to rule out the possibility of placenta previa (see p. 156) or of miscarriage.
● If you have had a previous miscarriage, ask your doctor's advice or ask at your prenatal clinic. You may be advised to abstain during the early months while the pregnancy establishes itself.
● If you have a show (see p. 173) or the waters break, there is a risk of infection.

POSITIONS FOR INTERCOURSE DURING PREGNANCY

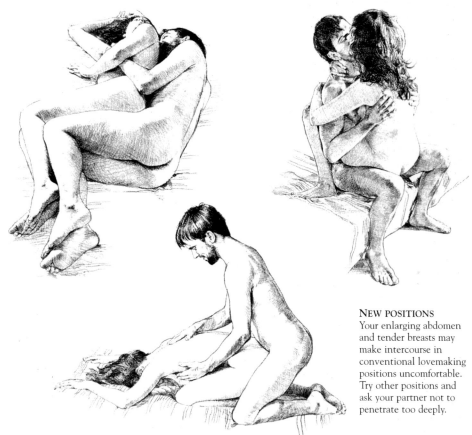

NEW POSITIONS
Your enlarging abdomen and tender breasts may make intercourse in conventional lovemaking positions uncomfortable. Try other positions and ask your partner not to penetrate too deeply.

8

Health and nutrition

To ensure that your baby develops in a healthy environment, you should keep your body as fit and well nourished as you possibly can. It's not a question of devising a special diet for pregnancy, it is more to do with eating a good variety of the right foods—those that are rich in the essential nutrients. If you are deficient in any part of your diet, this may affect not only your health but also how well you can support the pregnancy and nourish the baby. You also need to be aware of the risks posed by nicotine, alcohol and drugs as they can have a detrimental effect on the growth and well-being of the baby.

Weight gain

NOWADAYS IT IS KNOWN that you should gain a lot more weight in pregnancy than was thought healthy in the past. The amount of weight put on by women in pregnancy varies between 20 and 30 pounds (9–13.5 kg) with the most rapid gain usually between weeks 24 and 32. Your uterus, plus the baby, the placenta and the fluids will account for more than half of your total weight gain. You also manufacture more blood (see p. 98) and you lay down fat to prepare for lactation.

I would not want to encourage anyone to gain an excessive amount of weight, but dieting is not a good idea during pregnancy. It is much more important to eat a balanced and varied diet. A British study showed that there was a higher incidence of low-birthweight babies amongst those women who ate less than the recommended levels of calories, vitamins and minerals.

On the other hand, there is a lower incidence of physical and mental abnormalities, spontaneous abortions and neonatal deaths when mothers have relatively high weight gain (though not when they become obese) and babies are born heavier. It has also been shown that prolonged labors are directly related to the way in which the uterus has grown during pregnancy, and that in turn depends on how well nourished the mother has been.

EATING WELL
A balanced diet that includes plenty of fresh fruit and vegetables will keep you healthy during pregnancy.

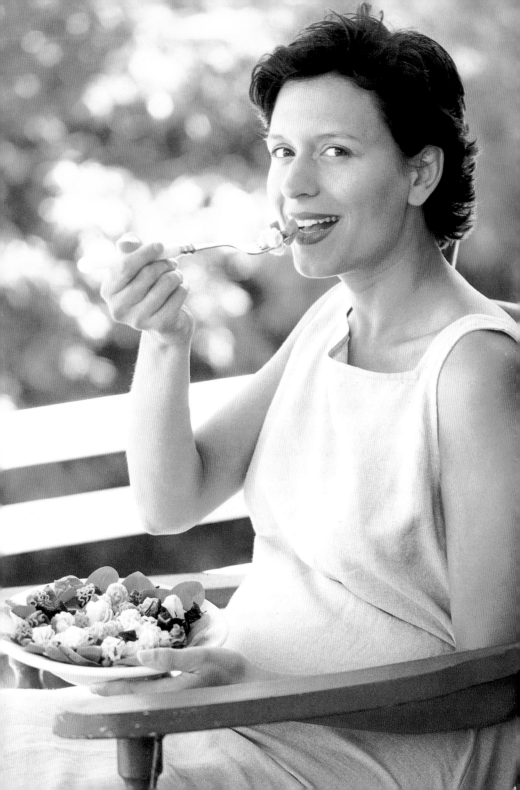

WHAT YOU GAIN

Rather than emphasizing restriction, nowadays doctors consider that minimum weight gain for most women should be 24 lb (11 kg). When a woman eats what she needs, her weight gain usually follows a natural and predictable pattern. You may find you put on weight and your figure changes almost from the time you confirm the pregnancy (6–8 weeks). However, your weight gain may be monitored from about 12 weeks at your prenatal checks.

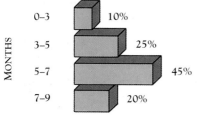

MONTHS

0–3	10%
3–5	25%
5–7	45%
7–9	20%

PERCENTAGE OF TOTAL WEIGHT GAIN
This is a rough guide to your weight gain at a given time during pregnancy.

BEING OVERWEIGHT

Although there is no ideal weight gain to aim for, it's still not a good idea for weight gain to be excessive. True obesity presents problems: it puts extra strain on the heart, which is already working at full stretch, and there is an association between excessive weight gain and cesarean section. It's thought that when fat accumulates between the muscle fibers of the uterus they work less efficiently and cannot contract enough to finish pushing the baby out once labor has started.

If you're definitely overweight and have been trying to lose weight, it's important that you stop dieting when you decide to try for a baby. Unless your doctor considers you are dangerously obese, choose your foods with care when you're trying to conceive and once you are pregnant, but don't do anything drastic about losing weight until you have finished breastfeeding your baby.

AWARENESS OF WEIGHT GAIN

If you run to plumpness during pregnancy, fat has a tendency to accumulate in places such as the thighs and upper arms. It is sometimes extremely difficult to lose this fat again after the birth. As this is demoralizing, here are a few tips to help you keep your weight gain within reasonable limits.

● As soon as you know that you are pregnant, get someone to take a snapshot of you, and take one every month or so after that. This reminder of your changing shape will help you keep your size in perspective, and if you feel you might be putting on too much weight, it may help you to combat cravings for foods with a high fat or sugar content.

● If you've always had a tendency to weight problems, but managed to keep them under control, it's easy to relapse into overeating once you know you're pregnant. Start eating sensibly from the beginning; try not to overeat in the first trimester when your appetite will almost certainly increase, even if you suffer from nausea some of the time.

● Try to eat regular, nutritious meals, and eat little and often when your pregnancy is more advanced. You're less likely to feel hungry in between.

● Keep a supply of nutritious snacks— cheese, fresh and dried fruit, wholemeal rolls—in the house and at your place of work at all times. Avoid the high calorie, low nutrition foods that are so accessible, such as candy bars, chips and soda.

● When preparing meals or snacks, follow these simple rules: eat unprocessed foods; include lots of roughage in your diet; grill rather than fry foods; sweeten with natural sweeteners.

● Don't eat as a way of cheering yourself up. If thinking about your baby and the birth makes you too distracted to concentrate on any serious project that would normally occupy you, at least have a project such as a jigsaw puzzle or a piece of embroidery to break up your routine.

GUIDELINES FOR EATING

Most of the daily food guides for pregnant women, with long lists of items to be prepared and measured out, don't take into account how busy most women are, or that they may not always be at home for meals. Rather than worry about exact portions, or lists, you should understand why you need certain foods and nutrients and work out your own plan for healthy eating. If you suffer from nausea, you may also have to plan when to prepare meals.

WHAT TO EAT

Your appetite will increase and by the fourth month of your pregnancy you may feel hungry all the time. This is nature's way of making sure that you take enough food for yourself and the baby. This doesn't mean you can "eat for two." It's perfectly normal to eat more as your metabolism speeds up, but your energy requirements increase only by about 15 percent, which means that 500 extra calories a day will be sufficient.

Every bit of food you take in should be good for you and the baby. If you ate well before you became pregnant, you should be healthy enough to get through any period of nausea (see p. 150). As your pregnancy progresses, try eating a greater number of smaller meals; small, frequent meals are always more easily digested. Bowel contractions slow down during pregnancy so the stomach empties more slowly and should not be overloaded at any one time. Your developing baby pushes up into your stomach during the last trimester, constricting its capacity, so a small meal is more easily accommodated and you'll feel more comfortable. The problem then arises of what sort of foods to eat as snacks. Avoid chips and cookies, which are usually low in goodness and high in calories. Be inventive, try sandwiches, nuts, fruit and soups.

FOODS TO AVOID

As a general rule, foods have a higher nutritional value the less they are processed and cooked. Choose fresh, raw wholefoods wherever you can. When planning what to eat, remember:
● Processed foods with added preservatives and colorings contain high levels of undesirable chemicals.
● White flour products or anything with added sugars provide little nutrition at the price of a lot of calories. Look at the list of ingredients on the labels of processed foods—you may be surprised how many apparently savory foods actually contain sugar!
● Sweet fizzy drinks—even if you choose the low calorie versions—are not good for you as they provide few nutrients and may contain harmful additives.
● Strong coffee and tea adversely affect the digestive system; tannic acid in tea drunk with a meal can reduce iron absorption. Excess caffeine and tannic acid may not be good for the baby.

● Certain foods may harbor dangerous bacteria and should be avoided during pregnancy: pâté and soft cheeses (listeria), raw eggs (salmonella).
● Liver or liver products should be eaten in moderation (see p. 114).
● Undercooked meat, unpasteurized goat's milk and goat's milk products may contain a parasite called toxoplasma, which can seriously harm the unborn baby. Only eat meat that has been cooked thoroughly. Avoid unpasteurized goat's milk and goat's milk products.
● Wash all fruits and vegetables thoroughly before eating or cooking to remove any traces of soil.
● Certain molds produce toxic substances so avoid eating fruits and vegetables with diseased skins, or any foods that are very moldy, or dried foods that are stale. It is not enough to remove the moldy parts as the harmful substances can penetrate deeper and they will not be destroyed by cooking.

Vital nutrients needed in pregnancy

YOU SHOULDN'T NEED to eat more food than you did before you were pregnant, but you should be aware of the nutrients present in the foods you choose to eat.

PROTEIN

Your protein requirements increase by about 50 percent when you are pregnant. In one day sufficient protein could be gained from three eggs, 1 pint (½ liter) milk, ¼ lb (100 g) cheese, or a good helping of fish or lean meat. These foods all contain the essential amino acids (the chemical substances that make up protein). Vegetable proteins contain only some of the amino acids so they need to be combined with animal protein or some wheat products to make them complete protein (see below). Vegetable proteins are found in peas, beans and lentils, brewer's yeast, seeds and nuts.

CALORIES

During pregnancy you will need about 500 more calories a day than the usual requirement of 2000–2500. You will need even more calories if you're having a baby within a short time of a previous one, or if you are still working, busy looking after a family, underweight or under stress. You shouldn't have to concentrate deliberately on calorie counting—most women are too busy to do this anyway—you will get sufficient calories if you eat a varied diet.

FIBER AND FLUIDS

As pregnancy progresses there is a tendency to develop constipation (see p. 148). You can help to overcome it by giving your intestines plenty of roughage to work on. Raw fruit and vegetables, bran, wholegrains, peas and beans are all fibrous foods that you should eat some of every day.

You should not regulate your fluid intake during pregnancy, except to watch the calorie content of the drinks you take. Water is the best drink, helping to keep your kidneys working well and to avoid constipation. If you do suffer from mild fluid retention (edema—see p. 152), you won't affect your condition by reducing your fluid intake.

VEGETARIAN DIET

Achieving a balanced diet with sufficient quantities of protein and all the vitamins and minerals doesn't require any more effort if you are a vegetarian. There are plant sources of protein that are complementary, so if you eat foods in combination you will gain all the necessary amino acids (see above). For example, if you are eating grains —rice or corn— combine them with dried beans or peas or nuts. If your meal is made up of fresh vegetables, add a few sesame seeds, nuts or mushrooms to supply the missing amino acids. Few people eat one food in isolation anyway. There is relatively little iron in each helping of plant food, even leafy green vegetables and beans, and these foods often contain substances that interfere with the body's absorption of iron, so vegetarians need to make sure that they eat plenty of foods that contain iron.

Pregnant vegetarians who don't take any dairy products (vegans) will need to be a little more careful that their diet is rich in foods that contain calcium, Vitamin D (or get plenty of sunshine) and riboflavin. The most difficult problem is adequate intake of vitamin B_{12}, which is only found in animal sources. Very little is needed but lack of it will lead to a form of anemia. It can be prepared commercially from fungi and you should consult your doctor about taking this synthetic B_{12} if you are a vegetarian.

VITAMINS

The value of a varied and balanced diet of wholesome food is that you will take in high enough levels of vitamins without resorting to vitamin supplements. Research has shown, however, that multivitamin supplements, if taken before conception and during the first trimester, can prevent neural tube defects such as anencephaly and spina bifida. There are other women who doctors consider may benefit from supplements (see below).

MINERALS

You are not likely to be deficient in minerals and trace elements if you eat a good diet. However, calcium and iron intakes need to be maintained and some doctors and clinics routinely prescribe dietary supplements of iron and folic acid. If supplements are not provided, ask if you need any. Your doctor may have assessed your diet and decided that it will be sufficient. Don't medicate yourself with supplements without your doctor knowing; discuss this with him or her first. Women who are nutritionally vulnerable, however, will certainly benefit from appropriate supplementation.

CALCIUM

A sufficient quantity of about twice your prepregnant intake is important from the time of conception because your baby's teeth and bones begin to form from weeks 4–6. As your baby grows, so your calcium requirements increase—by week 25 they have more than doubled. Sources of calcium include dairy foods, leafy vegetables, dried peas, beans and lentils, and nuts.

Calcium cannot be absorbed efficiently without Vitamin D. However, this vitamin is not found in great quantities in many foods and the best source is sunlight. The body can make its own vitamin D with the help of the sun so you don't need to worry about eating foods rich in vitamin D (butter, milk, egg yolk) unless you never expose your skin to sunlight.

Calcium supplements will be useful if you are allergic to cow's milk. You will need up to 1200 mg daily in a compound form, although if you eat well, 600 mg should be sufficient. Vitamin D will also be prescribed and is usually given in the form of halibut oil capsules which contain vitamin A as well.

IRON

The large increase in blood volume means that extra iron is needed to make hemoglobin for the increased number of red blood cells. The more hemoglobin the blood contains, the more oxygen it can carry to the various tissues, including the placenta. Your iron reserves will also be needed by the baby to have in reserve for after the birth, because breast milk contains only traces of iron.

Iron is quite difficult for the body to absorb. That from animal sources (prawns, egg yolk) is more easily absorbed than

NUTRITIONALLY VULNERABLE WOMEN

If any of the following apply to you, you need to make a special effort to eat well during pregnancy and will almost certainly need supplements to maintain your health and the general health of your baby.

● You are allergic to certain key foods, such as cow's milk or wheat.

● Before conception you were generally rundown, underweight or eating a poor and unbalanced diet.

● You have had a recent miscarriage or stillbirth, or your children are spaced closely together.

● You drink or smoke heavily.

● You have a chronic condition that obliges you to take some form of medication constantly.

● You are adolescent and still growing.

● You have a multiple pregnancy.

● For reasons beyond your control you have to work particularly hard or are subject to a lot of stress.

that in whole grains and nuts, but eating foods rich in vitamin C at the same time as those that are iron-rich can double the amount of iron absorbed.

If women are iron-deficient when they become pregnant or develop a deficiency later on, iron tablets may be prescribed to prevent anemia from developing (see p. 73).

There has been much unnecessary alarm about one iron-rich foodstuff, liver (and liver products). This is because cattle feeds are usually rich in vitamin A, which is concentrated in the animal's liver. Excessively large doses of vitamin A may carry a small risk to the baby of birth defects, so you should eat liver no more than once a week, in a small portion.

If you suffer from indigestion and take medication, be careful about your iron intake; antacid medicines limit iron absorption. Also, be aware that food cooked in iron pots absorbs iron, increasing the food's iron content by some three to 30 times.

VITAMINS AND MINERALS REQUIRED IN PREGNANCY

NAME	FOOD SOURCE	WHAT IT DOES
VITAMIN A (retinol)	whole milk, fortified margarine, butter, egg yolk, oily fish, fish liver oils, liver, kidneys, green and yellow vegetables, carrots—cooking the carrots releases vitamin A for easy absorption	Builds up resistance to infection, essential for good vision, keeps skin and mucous membranes in good condition, necessary for the formation of tooth enamel, hair and fingernails, important for the growth and formation of the thyroid gland.
VITAMIN B_1 (thiamine)	whole grains, nuts, liver, heart, kidneys, brewer's yeast, wheatgerm—don't overcook, benefits will be lost	Aids digestion, keeps the stomach and intestine healthy, needed for fertility, growth and lactation; the body's needs increase during illness and infection.
VITAMIN B_2 (riboflavin)	brewer's yeast, wheatgerm, whole grains, green vegetables, milk, eggs, liver—goodness can be lost if foods are exposed to light	Helps break down all food, prevents eye and skin problems, essential at the time of conception and early in pregnancy for normal development of the embryo.
NIACIN (B_3)	brewer's yeast, whole grains, liver, wheatgerm, green vegetables, oily fish, kidneys, eggs, milk, peanuts	Builds brain cells, prevents infections and bleeding of the gums.
PANTOTHENIC ACID (B_5)	liver, kidneys, heart, eggs, peanuts, wheatbran, whole grains, cheese	Essential for all normal reproductive functions of the body, maintains red blood cells.
VITAMIN B_6 (pyridoxine)	brewer's yeast, whole grains, liver, heart, kidneys, wheatgerm, mushrooms, potatoes, bananas, molasses, dried vegetables	Helps the body to assimilate fats and fatty acids necessary for the production of antibodies which fight disease; deficiency causes disease of the nerves and anemia.
VITAMIN B_{12} (cyanocobalamin)	liver, brewer's yeast, wheatgerm, whole grains, milk, soya beans, fish	Essential for the development of healthy red blood cells, necessary for the formation of the baby's central nervous system.
FOLIC ACID (one of B complex)	raw leaf vegetables, lamb's liver, walnuts	Essential for blood formation, helps to prevent neural tube defects, such as spina bifida; essential for the development of the central nervous system.

FOLIC ACID

Folic acid is essential for the supply of nucleic acids needed by the dividing cells of the embryo. As the body can't store folic acid and in pregnancy excretes four or five times the normal amount, enough must be eaten every day. Folic acid is found in leafy vegetables and nuts, but folic acid supplements should ideally be taken for three months before you become pregnant and throughout pregnancy (see p. 34).

Supplements of higher doses up to 4 mg may be prescribed for women who have previously had babies with brain and spinal cord defects such as spina bifida.

SALT

Ordinarily most of us take in too much sodium, but while you are pregnant, maintain a sensible salt intake. Any excess salt in your blood is diluted during pregnancy by the increase in body fluids.

NAME	FOOD SOURCE	WHAT IT DOES
VITAMIN C (ascorbic acid)	citrus fruits, fresh fruit, red, green and yellow vegetables—destroyed by overcooking	Helps resistance to infection, builds a strong placenta, helps the absorption of iron from the intestine, a useful detoxicant in the body, important for the repair of fractures and wound healing. Needs are variable; infection, fever and stress deplete the body's resources and needs increase.
VITAMIN D (calciferol)	fortified milk, oily fish, liver oils, butter, egg yolk—sunshine activates a previtamin in the skin (see p. 113)	Promotes the absorption of calcium from the intestine and helps the incorporation of calcium from the blood and tissues into bone cells to strengthen the bones.
VITAMIN E	wheatgerm, most other foods	Necessary for the healthy maintenance of cell membranes, also helps protect certain fatty acids.
VITAMIN K	green leafy vegetables— manufactured by the body from bacteria in the gut	Helps in the process by which blood coagulates.
CALCIUM	milk, hard cheese, whole small fish, peanuts, walnuts, sunflower seeds, green vegetables	Essential for the formation of healthy bones and teeth, important in the early months when the baby's teeth are developing.
IRON	kidneys, liver, shellfish, egg yolks, red meat, molasses, apricots, haricot beans, raisins, prunes	Essential for healthy formation of the red blood cells.
ZINC	wheatbran, eggs, liver, nuts, onions, shellfish, sunflower seeds, wheatgerm, whole wheat	Helps in formation of many enzymes (special proteins that oversee chemical reactions in our bodies) and of proteins, needed to ensure the release of vitamin A from liver stores into the bloodstream.

Handy foodstuffs

POTATOES ARE MUCH MALIGNED and underrated, but they are extremely nutritious, so do include them in your diet. A potato contains about 1 oz (3 g) of protein, together with calcium, iron, thiamin, riboflavin, and niacin, plus seven times as much vitamin C as an apple. If you don't want to add a lot of calories, don't fry them. Try to cook them in the skins, whether you are baking, boiling whole or mashing; peeling them first means you lose fiber, most of the protein, many of the vitamins and half the iron.

Another useful food is milk; it is easy to use, a cheap source of protein, and provides calcium together with vitamins A and D. The cream in milk contains half its calories and low-fat or skim milk, where the cream is removed, is preferable.

If you don't like drinking milk, use it on cereals, in custards, soups and sauces, or eat cheese (two small cubes of cheddar are equal to one small glass of milk) or yogurt. If you are allergic to milk, be careful to substitute other sources of the nutrients it provides, especially calcium (see p. 113).

You will see from the foods mentioned in this chapter that a few sources will provide the goodness you need for your own health and the development of your baby. Unless you are on a macrobiotic diet, your daily needs will be met by eating some of the following foodstuffs each day: milk or yogurt, eggs, fish, lean meat, offal (kidneys), yeast products, hard cheeses, whole grain foods (brown bread, pasta or rice), fresh fruit and vegetables, fruit juices, nuts, dried fruits.

DIET AND MORNING SICKNESS

Ironically women who suffer from nausea in the first three months of pregnancy can be hungry at the same time. Food provides relief from the nausea, though the nausea soon returns. To combat this, many women find that small, frequent snacks and an avoidance of the trigger foods (usually rich, creamy or spicy foods) and smells (cigarette smoke, frying food) can help during the difficult weeks. Though called morning sickness, nausea can occur at any time of the day or even throughout the day. Work out your "good" times and prepare your meals and snacks then.

Eating more starch does seem to alleviate the sick feeling. However, this can also lead to excessive weight gain. Fat does need to be laid down in the first trimester (see p. 108), so if it's a question of eating carbohydrate in the form of a bun or cake, it's better to eat that than nothing at all, especially if you are vomiting. There are more nutritious forms of carbohydrate such as wholemeal bread, rice and potatoes, so eat these rather than sweets, cakes and iced buns.

Here are some snacks you can prepare at home or have at your workplace:
- slices of dried wholegrain bread
- wholegrain-bread cheese sandwiches
- nuts and raisins
- dried apricots
- fruit cake (preferably made with wholegrain flour and wheatgerm added)
- green crisp apples
- water crackers and cottage cheese
- raw vegetables such as carrots, celery, tender young green beans, peas from the pod, tomatoes
- diluted fresh fruit juices
- carbonated water with a slice of lemon
- bitter lemon or lime
- diabetic peppermints sucked slowly
- commercial muesli bars with bran, coconut or apple added
- unflavored, natural yogurt with honey
- fruit sorbet
- herbal teas
- soft, juicy fruits such as peaches, plums and pears
- milkshakes made with skim milk.

Dangerous substances

IF YOU NORMALLY SMOKE or drink, you should change your habits during pregnancy to protect your unborn baby. You also need to be meticulous about hygiene, particularly when handling raw meat and when cleaning out cat litter. Raw meat and cat feces contain a parasite, toxoplasma, that can damage your unborn child.

SMOKING

● The chemicals absorbed from cigarette smoke limit fetal growth by reducing the number of cells produced, both in the baby's body and brain. Nicotine makes blood vessels constrict and therefore reduces the blood supply to the placenta, interfering with the nourishment of the baby.
● The level of carbon monoxide is higher in a smoker's blood, and whatever the level in the woman's blood it's higher in the baby's blood. As well as being a poison, carbon monoxide reduces the amount of oxygen that blood can carry. The more carbon monoxide in the baby's blood, the lower its weight at birth. The babies of mothers who smoke can be as much as 7 oz (200 g) lighter than those of mothers who don't smoke, and low birthweight babies can have problems and are less likely to survive. The incidence of prematurity almost doubles in smokers.
● Studies have shown that smokers are more likely to have children with all types of congenital malformations, especially cleft palate, hare lip and central nervous system abnormalities, with the risk more than doubled in heavy smokers.
● Smokers have nearly twice the risk of spontaneous abortion (miscarriage and stillbirth), partly because smoking greatly increases the risk of the placenta being attached too low down in the uterus (see p. 156), and partly because smokers' placentas tend to be thinner and age prematurely.
● Neonatal deaths are more common among babies whose mothers smoked.

Mothers who continue to smoke after the fourth month are increasing by nearly one third the risk of their baby dying.
● The effects of smoking in pregnancy last for a long time after your baby is born, and children who live in smoking households are less healthy than others in many respects. Exposure to cigarette smoke puts babies at considerable risk during the first year of life—they have a tendency to develop bronchitis and the incidence of crib deaths increases.

HOW MUCH?

While all smoking is thought to be harmful, the death rate in smokers' babies tends to tail off below ten cigarettes a day. Women

---

TIPS TO CUT DOWN SMOKING

You may be finding it difficult to give up smoking during pregnancy, so here are some tips to help you cut down and then to stop:
● cut down to less than ten a day
● only smoke the lowest tar and nicotine brand of cigarette
● always smoke filter tips
● stop inhaling
● put out a long stub—most of the nicotine and tar is in the second half of the cigarette
● if you smoke out of nervousness, occupy your hands with something else, such as worry beads
● if you need to feel something in your mouth, chew sugar-free gum (try to avoid sucking sweets, eating more or drinking lots of tea and coffee)
● avoid nicotine gum or patches; the nicotine will still cross the placenta to the baby, even if you avoid some of the other 3000 toxic chemicals in cigarette smoke
● watch your diet: smokers may be deficient in zinc, manganese, vitamins A, B_6, B_{12}, and C.

who cut down on cigarettes or stop smoking before week 20 tend to have babies of a similar birthweight to nonsmokers, but that still leaves the risk of congenital abnormality caused by smoking in the early stages, or even before conception (see p. 35). Women who live with smokers or are often in a smoky environment are at risk even if they never smoke themselves. Children of fathers who smoke heavily are twice as likely to have malformations.

It's particularly important that a woman who is in need of special care during pregnancy for any reason doesn't smoke because she is adding a factor that increases the possibility of something going wrong. So, if a woman has suffered a stillbirth, it is crucial that she doesn't smoke the next time she becomes pregnant as this would multiply her chances of another stillbirth.

DRINKING ALCOHOL

The extent to which alcohol, a poison, can seriously damage a developing baby has only been appreciated in the last ten or so years. Some of the alcohol of every drink you take reaches your baby's bloodstream and is most harmful during the critical development period of weeks 6–12, although each affected growth period seems to produce its own abnormalities.

There is no safe level of alcohol consumption in pregnancy. If you have more than two drinks a day, there is a one in ten chance that your baby will have fetal alcohol syndrome (FAS), which can lead to facial abnormalities such as cleft palate and hare lip, heart defects, abnormal limb development and lower than average intelligence. Seriously affected babies never catch up mentally or physically with their counterparts. Binge-drinking can cause the same damage, even if you drink little as a rule: one incident of excessive alcohol consumption is just as capable of giving rise to FAS as drinking excessively all through pregnancy. You should, therefore, limit yourself to two glasses of

spirits or wine, or 1 pint (570 ml) of beer on any one day. Some studies show that babies can be affected in less severe ways by intakes below two glasses a day. Perhaps this is because some mothers metabolize alcohol into poisonous acetaldehyde very quickly, perhaps because some babies are genetically less resistant to the effects of alcohol—as yet no one knows. It has been demonstrated that as little as one drink a day can double the risk of having an underweight baby, and babies of women drinking half that amount tend to be shorter than expected. It is beginning to be thought that very small intakes of alcohol can cause many mental conditions so far unexplained, or affect babies mentally and physically in subtle ways. In the present state of knowledge, it would seem sensible for women once they decide to have a child, not to drink at all (see p. 35) and to abstain from drinking alcohol throughout the pregnancy.

DRUGS

It's well known that certain drugs can affect the development of a baby, particularly at the sensitive period between weeks 6 and 12 when all the vital organs are being formed. In addition a drug may be safe in itself, but it can be harmful to the fetus if taken in combination with another equally innocent drug or certain foods.

Because of these dangers *no drug of any kind, and that includes aspirin, should be taken unless under the supervision of a doctor.* Don't take over-the-counter remedies for anything, or use leftover prescription drugs, or accept drugs prescribed for other people. And don't consult a doctor about anything without informing him or her that you are pregnant or trying to become pregnant.

Some drugs have to be taken for the treatment of chronic complaints (see p. 37) such as diabetes, heart disease, thyroid problems, rheumatic disorders and possibly epilepsy, but discuss the continuation of medication with your doctor before you conceive.

EFFECTS OF DRUGS ON YOUR BABY

DRUG NAME	EFFECTS
AMPHETAMINES	They are stimulants in adults and also stimulate the baby's nervous system. They may cause heart defects and blood diseases. Sometimes present in diet pills.
ANABOLIC STEROIDS	These are related to male sex hormones. They have a masculinizing effect on a female fetus. May be present in treatments for hay fever or skin disorders. May be present in ointments prescribed for skin irritation—avoid during pregnancy.
ANTIBIOTICS	They do cross the placenta but penicillin would seem to be safe.
TETRACYCLINE	Used for long-term treatment of acne. Avoid because it causes permanent yellow discoloration of the baby's teeth and may interfere with growth of bones and teeth.
STREPTOMYCIN	May cause deafness in infants. It is used to treat tuberculosis.
ANTIHISTAMINES	Treat allergic reactions; may be prescribed for morning sickness. Present in some travel sickness drugs. May cause malformations so only use with medical supervision.
ANTI-NAUSEA DRUGS	Some of them have been shown to produce malformation in animal testing. It's better to try to combat nausea through your diet (see p. 116). If your nausea is very severe, your doctor will know of a safe drug.
ASPIRIN	May be given by your doctor for pre-eclampsia (see p. 162) or poor fetal growth. However, excessive amounts may cause miscarriage so it should only be taken under medical supervision.
BIRTH CONTROL PILLS estrogen/ progesterone	Can cause malformations of the limbs, defects of the vital organs and masculinization of the female fetus. Better to stop taking the pill at least three months before conceiving (see p. 38).
CODEINE	Used in pain relief and in some cough medicines. Increased incidence of malformations, such as cleft palate and hare lip, have been reported. Is an addictive drug, can cause withdrawal symptoms in the baby at birth.
DIURETICS	These are used to get rid of excess fluid from the body. They make your kidneys work harder. They can cause some blood disorders in the fetus.
PARACETAMOL	A common ingredient of cold remedies and painkillers. Used with caution it is generally regarded as safe, but in excess can damage the fetus's kidneys and liver.
PROGESTOGENS	Given by mouth may cause fetal malformation. May be used as a treatment for recurrent miscarriage, but administered as pessaries or suppositories.
STREET DRUGS	Some cause chromosomal damage, others may cause fetal addiction. Little is known about the effects of many "recreational" drugs, so avoid them altogether.
SULFONAMIDES	Can disturb the developing baby's liver function and cause jaundice at birth. Used to treat urinary infections.
TRANQUILIZERS	Some of the stronger types may affect growth and development, causing malformations. Consult your doctor about changing to a milder tranquilizer but try to do without for the duration of your pregnancy.

9

Exercise

Both before and during pregnancy, exercise is essential. Before pregnancy, it ensures that your body is fit to carry a healthy baby to term. Once pregnant, it strengthens muscles to protect your joints and spine, which slacken prior to labor and ache when overused. Specific exercises, when combined with breathing and relaxation techniques, help conserve energy in labor, while others prepare you for delivery positions.

Being aware of your body

YOUR BODY CHANGES in many ways during pregnancy. There are the obvious physical changes (see pp. 92–101), as well as the loosening up and stretching of the ligaments around the joints. But more important, on a day-to-day basis, is the difference in what your body can do with ease compared to what it could before.

In later pregnancy you become a rather ungainly shape and lose some agility and mobility, becoming breathless more easily. Your center of gravity is further forward and you are less stable. Once committed to a certain direction you may find it hard to change, and if someone bumps into you, you may fall over. To compensate for this lack of stability, you might hold your shoulders back, stand with your feet apart, and walk with a waddling gait.

These compensatory actions mean that you are using muscles in a different way and may therefore suffer minor aches and pains as pregnancy progresses. If, however, you keep your body fit during pregnancy, and protect it from stresses and strains, the muscles, joints and ligaments will take the strain more easily, without aching. You may even avoid minor discomforts

altogether. Get used to thinking that your body is in a special, not an abnormal, state, and develop reflexes and postures that take account of its needs. If you do feel uncomfortable, ease your discomfort with relaxation techniques (see p. 143).

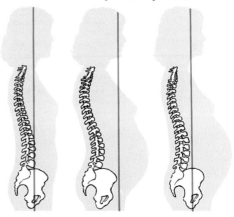

CORRECTING BAD POSTURE
Your center of gravity (left) is affected by the growing baby in pregnancy when there is a tendency to lean back to compensate for the increased weight (center). Good posture (right) corrects your balance and helps avoid aches.

BENDING AND LIFTING

The hormones of pregnancy soften the ligaments of the lower back and pelvis so heavy lifting should be avoided. You must protect your spine at this time and avoid unnecessary strain on your lower back when bending or lifting.

Make use of your thigh muscles when lifting. Squat down first, keeping your back straight. Prepare your body (keep your feet slightly apart) by tensing the abdominal muscles, pulling up your pelvic floor muscles (see p. 124), taking a deep breath and counting to three before lifting on four. As you lift, breathe out. Stand close to whatever you are lifting and keep it close to your body as you pick it up.

• When you are carrying anything, avoid swiveling to either side and try to distribute the weight evenly, as for instance with heavy shopping baskets.

• When you are carrying your toddler keep your body straight, don't twist, and change him from side to side.

• If you have to do anything that involves being low down, squat (see p. 131) or get down on all fours. This is a comfortable position, particularly if you do suffer from backache, as it takes the weight of the uterus off your spine.

If you have bad posture, or your back isn't flexible, improve your suppleness by sitting cross-legged against a wall. Lengthen your spine, and tilt your pelvis, pressing your back into the wall. This helps to strengthen your spine and shows you how to hold yourself well.

• Avoid lifting anything heavy down from a height. Your back will arch and you could lose your balance if the object is heavier than you supposed.

PROTECTING YOUR SPINE

In later pregnancy you will need to adapt all your movements, even basic everyday ones like getting up from lying down or getting out of a chair. You want to put the least strain possible on your back and let your thighs do the work.

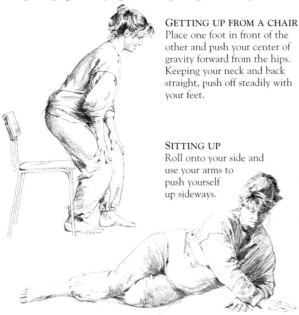

GETTING UP FROM A CHAIR
Place one foot in front of the other and push your center of gravity forward from the hips. Keeping your neck and back straight, push off steadily with your feet.

SITTING UP
Roll onto your side and use your arms to push yourself up sideways.

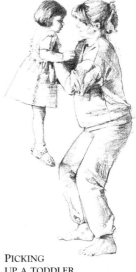

PICKING UP A TODDLER
Remember to keep your back straight and to bend your knees.

Keeping active

PREGNANCY, LABOR AND DELIVERY will make great demands on your body, so the more you can prepare yourself physically, the better. Whether you do this by continuing to exercise in the way you did before pregnancy (see p. 132) or whether you embark on a new form of exercise is up to you. The important thing is to keep yourself active. The fitter you are, the less likelihood there will be of your stiffening up as pregnancy progresses. If you make sure that you sit, stand and walk in the correct ways (see p. 121), you should avoid the aches and pains that invariably come with bad posture.

THE BENEFITS OF BEING FIT

Regular exercise will improve your mental as well as your physical well-being. Exercise causes the body to release tranquillizing chemicals, helping you to relax and soothing away tensions and anxiety. And the fast circulation of the blood that occurs when you exercise means that your body and your baby are well oxygenated.

Labor will almost certainly be easier and more comfortable if you have good muscle tone, and many of the exercises taught in prenatal classes, combined with relaxation and breathing techniques, will help give you more control over what is happening to you.

Keeping in condition during pregnancy will also mean that you regain your normal shape more quickly after delivery, and regular exercise of the pelvic floor muscles (see p. 125) will not only assist in delivery, but will also allow the muscles to regain their normal strength more quickly.

However, before you start on any exercise program in early pregnancy, check with your doctor to make sure it is safe. Some doctors feel that if a woman has a history of miscarriage or there are any complications she should not undertake exercises in the first three months of pregnancy.

When you have the "all-clear," here are a few tips for keeping fit:
- Try to enroll in an exercise class specially designed for pregnant women. Many women find it easier to exercise regularly this way as they have the discipline of a teacher putting them through the exercises. It also helps to have someone watching you, correcting the way in which the exercises are done.
- If you haven't been an active person before pregnancy you're unlikely to change dramatically during it, but at least try to walk whenever you can, 20 minutes a day if you can manage it.
- Even if you have to sit down all day, there are exercises that you can do in a chair (see p. 129).
- Get into the habit of going through a 10–15 minute exercise program every day. During pregnancy, exercises should be regular and taken at a slow pace. They should be rhythmic whenever possible, so it's a good idea to exercise to music.
- Always warm up gently before you start your exercise program (see p. 126).
- Try not to go for periods with no exercise at all. Even a little exercise several times a day is better than a big burst followed by a long gap.
- Never exercise to the point of fatigue.
- Never do an exercise that causes you pain. Pain is a signal that something is wrong. Try a simpler variation of the exercise. Work towards a position gradually, don't strain.
- Try not to point your toes for too long when you're exercising as it may cause cramps in the legs.
- Most exercises are done on the floor and you might like to have a few pillows or cushions as aids to make yourself comfortable.
- Before each exercise, try a few deep breaths. This is relaxing, it makes you feel alert, it gets the blood flowing around your body and gives all your muscles a good supply of oxygen.

Prenatal exercise classes

A VARIETY OF PRENATAL exercise classes are available and it is worth doing some research into what they have to offer and what type of teaching you'd be happiest with. The hospital or clinic will run classes (see p. 71) or you can go to an independent organization or a workshop specially for pregnant women (see p. 244 for addresses of organizations).

WHAT THEY TEACH

Some classes are run just like an ordinary exercise class, giving a thorough physical workout with exercises specifically designed for pregnant women to increase flexibility, strength and stamina. Others are designed with a certain philosophy of birth in mind. If you want to give birth in a squatting position, there will be exercises to strengthen the back and thighs, for example. The classes are also good places for making contact with other pregnant women.

YOGA

With its emphasis on muscular control of the body, breathing, relaxation and tranquillity of mind, yoga is an excellent method to use as a preparation for pregnancy. However, yoga is a philosophy which pervades the whole of life and, though special exercises for pregnancy exist, they are only a small part of the system. If you are already a devotee or have made the effort to become familiar with yoga-based exercises prior to your pregnancy, yoga can be of great help in increasing your sense of well-being. Yoga exercises are comparable with some of those taught in prenatal classes but the types of breathing used are different. It is believed that these breathing techniques help to raise the pain threshold.

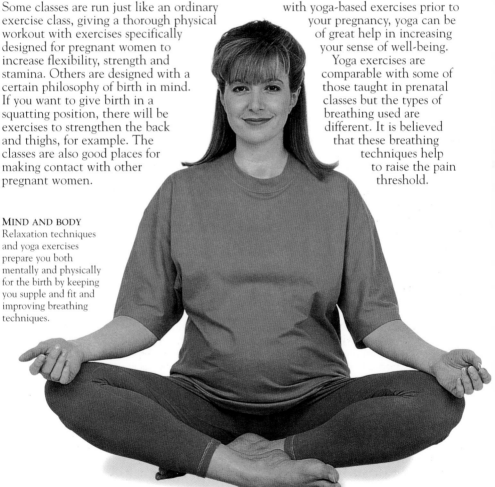

MIND AND BODY
Relaxation techniques and yoga exercises prepare you both mentally and physically for the birth by keeping you supple and fit and improving breathing techniques.

The pelvic floor muscles

THE MUSCLES THAT MAKE UP the pelvic floor support the uterus, bowel and bladder, rather like a sling holding the pelvic organs in place. They lie in two main groups, forming a figure of eight around the urethra, vagina and anus. The muscle fibers originate front and back from high up on the pubic and sacral bones. The layers of muscle overlap and are therefore thickest at the perineum.

THE ACTION OF PROGESTERONE

The pregnancy hormone progesterone prepares the body for birth by softening joints and ligaments, and that includes the pelvic floor muscles. If pressure from the enlarging uterus causes the pelvic floor to become weak, this can lead to vague aches and fatigue, to urinary incontinence and leakage, and possibly, at worst, even to prolapse of the uterus after childbirth. About half the women who have had children subsequently suffer from some weakness of the pelvic floor. As a result they may experience discomfort or so-called "stress" incontinence—slight leakage of urine when they laugh, cough, sneeze, or lift.

To counter this, a set of exercises to strengthen the pelvic floor muscles has been developed by physiotherapists working in the area of childbirth. They are known as the Kegel exercises, after Dr. Arnold Kegel of the University of California in Los Angeles, one of the first physicians to recognize how important these muscles are.

Pelvic floor exercises are recommended for all women. It's best to begin doing the exercises before pregnancy and continue afterwards (they are probably even more important in older women). If you possibly can, make the exercises (see opposite) part of your daily routine.

When exercising, do about five contractions of five seconds each. Once you've mastered the exercises, you can do them wherever you are—sitting at home, standing in a queue or walking—but do remember to practice as often as you can. They will also be useful in the second stage of labor when the baby's head is about to be born (see opposite below).

LOCATING THE PELVIC FLOOR MUSCLES

Lie down with a pillow under your head and one under your knees. Cross one leg over the other and squeeze your legs tightly together. Tighten the buttock muscles and pull up as if you feel the need to empty your bladder but must wait. This helps you to locate the pelvic floor muscles, which you will feel tighten inside your vagina.

Another way to locate the muscles is to interrupt the flow midstream when you pass urine, because the muscles that control the flow of urine are your pelvic floor muscles. Always make sure that you empty your bladder completely after stopping the flow of urine several times. When doing the exercises (see opposite), ignore the abdominal and buttock muscles and use only those of the pelvic floor.

ISOLATING THE SPHINCTER MUSCLES

Lie down as above but with your legs relaxed and not crossed. Place a clean fingertip on the opening of your vagina and contract your pelvic floor muscles. You will be able to feel the contraction of the vaginal sphincter. The sphincter at the opening of the urethra is more difficult to isolate than the pelvic floor muscles because of its proximity to the vagina. But the sphincter muscles are also tightened when you contract the pelvic floor muscles.

Now place your finger at the opening of your bowels and, with a larger movement, contract the muscle around the anus. You will feel the anal sphincter tightening.

STRENGTHENING THE PELVIC FLOOR

During pregnancy, the increase in the hormone progesterone causes the pelvic floor muscles to soften and relax. Here are three basic Kegel exercises which will help you to strengthen your pelvic floor muscles and keep them well toned during pregnancy. You should try to make these exercises part of your daily routine before, as well as during, pregnancy and then start them again as soon as possible after the delivery to minimize the risk of prolapse.

Contract and release

Lie on your back with your legs apart. Draw up the pelvic floor muscles, concentrating hard on the muscles of the vaginal sphincter. Hold this position for two to three seconds and then completely relax. You can try to slacken the muscles a little more and notice the release in tension. Do three of these contractions in succession.

The lift

Imagine the pelvic floor is a lift, stopping at various levels in a department store. Aim to contract the muscles gradually in five stages with a short stop at each level, not letting go between levels. Then allow the pelvic floor to descend, releasing the contraction level by level. When you reach the starting point, ground level, allow the pelvic floor muscles to relax completely so that you feel a slight bulging downwards. If you actually push downwards below this level, as if sending the elevator into the basement, you can lower the pelvic floor even further, and the vaginal lips will open slightly. To do this, however, you need to hold your breath or blow out and then you should be able to feel the lips of the vaginal opening. Remember, this is the position in which your pelvic floor should be if you have an internal examination and while your baby's head is being born.

During sex

Grip your partner's penis with your vagina. Hold for a few seconds before releasing. Repeat this exercise a couple of times. Your partner will be able to tell you how hard you are squeezing and will know when the strength of the squeeze is diminishing. If your partner says that he can't feel much, then you will know that you must keep exercising your pelvic muscles.

PREPARING FOR THE BIRTH OF THE BABY'S HEAD

Having an increased awareness of the pelvic floor muscles and how they feel when relaxed will help prepare you for the birth of your baby's head.

Exercise one

Lie on a bed with your knees bent, feet together and your back supported. Press your knees together hard and tighten the pelvic floor muscles at the same time. Note the feeling of tension along the inner thighs and between your legs; many women involuntarily tense these muscles when their baby's head is stretching the outlet of the birth canal, and in fact you should try to avoid this because you are more likely to tense up during delivery. Relax, and notice carefully the different feel of the muscles; this open feeling is what you should aim for when giving birth.

Exercise two

Lie on a bed, your back supported, but with your feet and knees apart. Gradually relax your thighs and pelvic floor muscles so that your knees fall wider and wider apart (your feet will roll gently onto their outer edges). At first this may seem somewhat unnatural and uncomfortable but after a little practice you will get the correct feeling of letting go fully. Practice panting in this position as you will be asked to do this by the midwife when it is time for your baby's head to pass slowly and gently out of the birth canal.

Stretching

ALWAYS PRECEDE your exercise program by warming up with these few stretching exercises. They gently warm up muscles and joints so that you can move more freely, reducing the risk of overstretching and damage. Warming up before exercising will also reduce the risk of suffering from stiffness and cramp. Furthermore, these exercises help to stimulate the circulation, giving you

and your baby a good supply of oxygen. Repeat each exercise five to ten times; work on a firm surface, make sure you are comfortable and that your posture is good with your back straight. If necessary, lean your back against a wall or use cushions for extra support. Remembering to breathe normally throughout, start the routine slowly and if you feel any pain, discomfort or fatigue, stop at once.

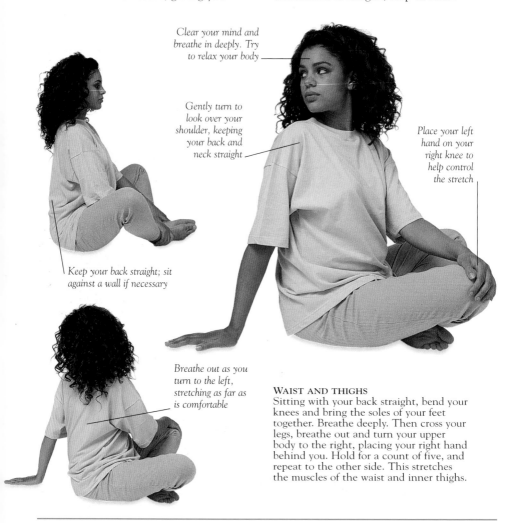

Clear your mind and breathe in deeply. Try to relax your body

Gently turn to look over your shoulder, keeping your back and neck straight

Place your left hand on your right knee to help control the stretch

Keep your back straight; sit against a wall if necessary

Breathe out as you turn to the left, stretching as far as is comfortable

WAIST AND THIGHS
Sitting with your back straight, bend your knees and bring the soles of your feet together. Breathe deeply. Then cross your legs, breathe out and turn your upper body to the right, placing your right hand behind you. Hold for a count of five, and repeat to the other side. This stretches the muscles of the waist and inner thighs.

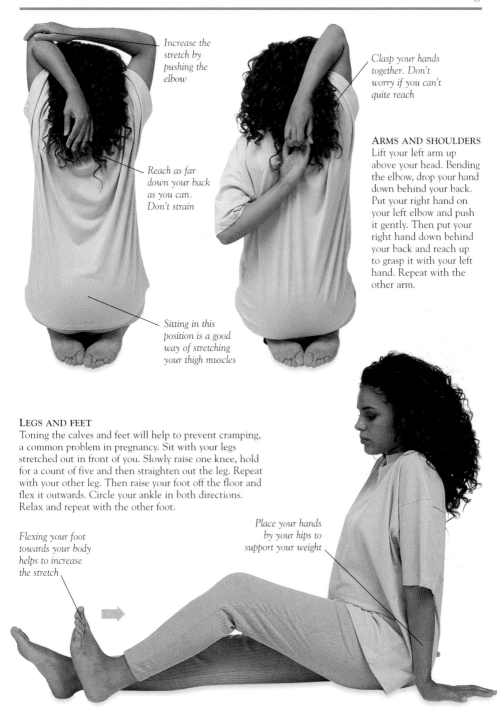

Increase the stretch by pushing the elbow

Clasp your hands together. Don't worry if you can't quite reach

Reach as far down your back as you can. Don't strain

ARMS AND SHOULDERS
Lift your left arm up above your head. Bending the elbow, drop your hand down behind your back. Put your right hand on your left elbow and push it gently. Then put your right hand down behind your back and reach up to grasp it with your left hand. Repeat with the other arm.

Sitting in this position is a good way of stretching your thigh muscles

LEGS AND FEET
Toning the calves and feet will help to prevent cramping, a common problem in pregnancy. Sit with your legs stretched out in front of you. Slowly raise one knee, hold for a count of five and then straighten out the leg. Repeat with your other leg. Then raise your foot off the floor and flex it outwards. Circle your ankle in both directions. Relax and repeat with the other foot.

Flexing your foot towards your body helps to increase the stretch

Place your hands by your hips to support your weight

Floor exercises

STRETCHING DIFFERENT PARTS of the body relieves strain and tones important muscles. Strengthening your lower back is particularly important, helping to prevent backache. By working on a firm surface and carrying out all movements smoothly, you shouldn't feel discomfort or strain. These exercises can easily be fitted into your day. Repeat each one five times to begin with, increasing slowly until you are doing 10 or 15. Don't, however, do these exercises after week 32 of pregnancy. At this late stage it's not a good idea to lie flat on your back for any length of time as the pressure of the uterus on deep veins in your pelvis may result in fainting and dizziness.

PELVIC LIFT

Lie flat on the floor with your arms by your sides. Pressing your feet into the floor, squeeze your buttocks and lift your pelvis up into the air as high as you can. Hold for a count of five. Gradually lower your back down one vertebra at a time.

Inhale, then breathe out as you raise your pelvis

Relax and don't hold your breath

Lower your back slowly, letting your thigh muscles do the work

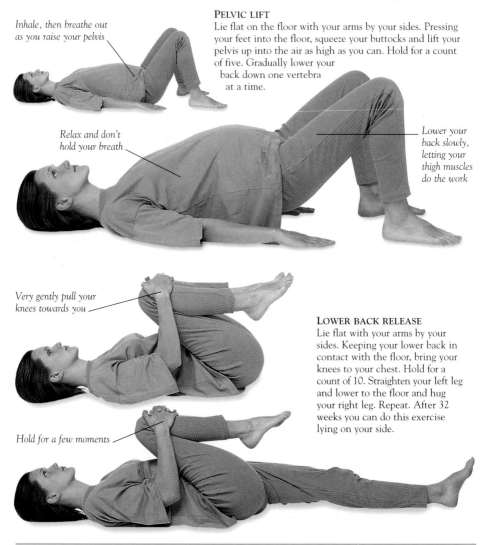

Very gently pull your knees towards you

LOWER BACK RELEASE

Lie flat with your arms by your sides. Keeping your lower back in contact with the floor, bring your knees to your chest. Hold for a count of 10. Straighten your left leg and lower to the floor and hug your right leg. Repeat. After 32 weeks you can do this exercise lying on your side.

Hold for a few moments

SITTING EXERCISES

It's easy to neglect parts of the body like the neck or the ankles. These stretches will keep you supple and help prevent the build-up of fluid (edema) that causes puffiness. You can do them anywhere: try them in the evening as you watch TV.

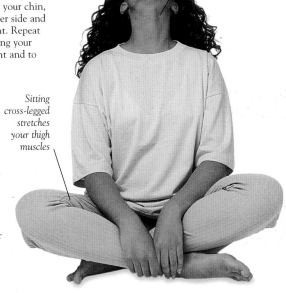

Rotate your neck slowly and carefully to avoid injury

HEAD AND NECK

Sit on the floor with your legs crossed and gently tilt your head over to one side. Lifting your chin, rotate your head back, over to the other side and down in one gentle, flowing movement. Repeat in the opposite direction. Then, keeping your head straight, turn it slowly to the right and to the left. Return to face the front.

ANKLES

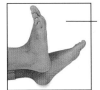

Circle 5 times to the left and then to the right

Sitting cross-legged stretches your thigh muscles

Sit barefoot on the floor with your legs outstretched in front of you. Raise your right leg slightly off the ground and draw large circles in the air using only your ankles. Put your foot back on the floor and repeat with your left ankle.

Only raise your hips a little way up from the floor

Relax your jaw. Concentrate on breathing evenly

HIP CIRCLING

Lie flat on the floor with your arms by your sides, palms down. Bend both knees and cross your feet at the ankles. Then rotate your hips clockwise, making tiny circles with your lower back on the floor. Relax and then repeat the movement in the opposite direction.

Use your arms to steady yourself

Twisting and bending

PREGNANCY HORMONES soften your ligaments in preparation for the birth; unfortunately they can also make you susceptible to strains and backache. Twisting and bending exercises help to strengthen key muscles, as well as to loosen up the pelvis in preparation for the birth. Getting down on all fours is an excellent way to ease backache, especially if you combine it with a few pelvic tilts.

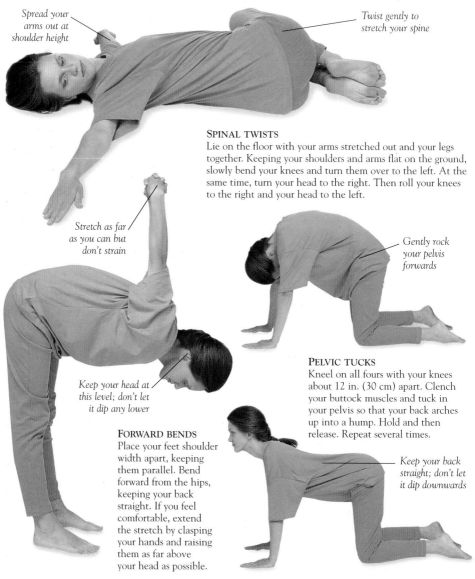

Spread your arms out at shoulder height

Twist gently to stretch your spine

SPINAL TWISTS
Lie on the floor with your arms stretched out and your legs together. Keeping your shoulders and arms flat on the ground, slowly bend your knees and turn them over to the left. At the same time, turn your head to the right. Then roll your knees to the right and your head to the left.

Stretch as far as you can but don't strain

Gently rock your pelvis forwards

Keep your head at this level; don't let it dip any lower

PELVIC TUCKS
Kneel on all fours with your knees about 12 in. (30 cm) apart. Clench your buttock muscles and tuck in your pelvis so that your back arches up into a hump. Hold and then release. Repeat several times.

FORWARD BENDS
Place your feet shoulder width apart, keeping them parallel. Bend forward from the hips, keeping your back straight. If you feel comfortable, extend the stretch by clasping your hands and raising them as far above your head as possible.

Keep your back straight; don't let it dip downwards

SQUATTING

There are many benefits to be derived from doing squatting exercises. Squatting cuts off some blood from the general circulation and so gives the heart a rest. It makes your joints, especially the pelvic ones, more flexible, stretches and strengthens the thighs and back muscles and relieves back pain. Squatting is a comfortable position to relax in and is a practical position for labor and delivery (see p. 183). It may seem difficult at first but with practice it will become progressively easier.

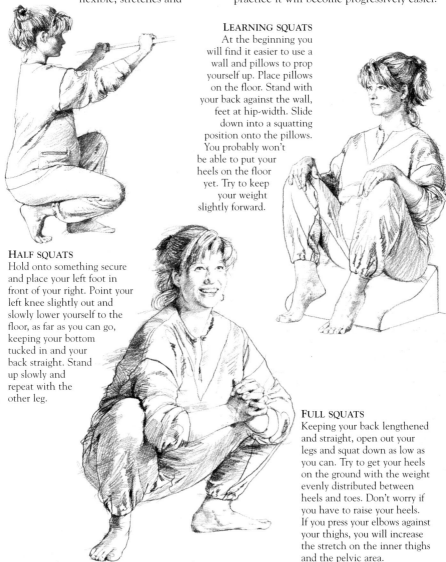

LEARNING SQUATS
At the beginning you will find it easier to use a wall and pillows to prop yourself up. Place pillows on the floor. Stand with your back against the wall, feet at hip-width. Slide down into a squatting position onto the pillows. You probably won't be able to put your heels on the floor yet. Try to keep your weight slightly forward.

HALF SQUATS
Hold onto something secure and place your left foot in front of your right. Point your left knee slightly out and slowly lower yourself to the floor, as far as you can go, keeping your bottom tucked in and your back straight. Stand up slowly and repeat with the other leg.

FULL SQUATS
Keeping your back lengthened and straight, open out your legs and squat down as low as you can. Try to get your heels on the ground with the weight evenly distributed between heels and toes. Don't worry if you have to raise your heels. If you press your elbows against your thighs, you will increase the stretch on the inner thighs and the pelvic area.

Sports activities

THERE ARE SEVERAL SPORTS that you can do as long as you take it gently and stop if you feel tired. Remember, if you are out of breath, your baby is deprived of oxygen.

WALKING

You can walk as much as you like—it's very good exercise. The main concern is that you walk under safe conditions.

SWIMMING

Swimming is an excellent form of exercise and the one sport you can continue until term. I swam two weeks before delivery with my second pregnancy, slowly and gently of course. Don't swim if the water is cold as you are more prone to cramping.

CYCLING AND DANCING

Cycling is good exercise, but stop when your abdomen gets so large that it starts to affect your center of gravity, as you might lose your balance. As long as you're not too energetic, you can dance throughout pregnancy. It is a good way to practice pelvic tilts.

SPORTS TO AVOID

Don't go riding or skiing during pregnancy. Even if you are experienced you could fall. The risks are too great.

TAKING THE WEIGHT
As well as improving your stamina, swimming supports your weight and helps you to relax.

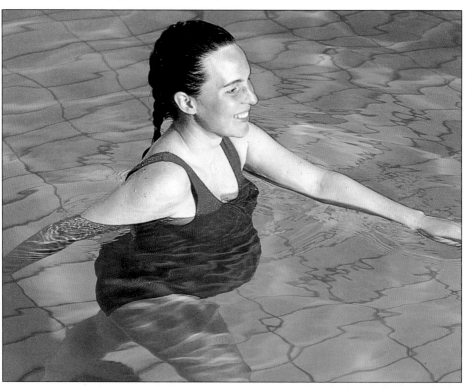

WATER EXERCISES

Swimming is wonderful exercise during pregnancy. You can improve your general fitness, while becoming more supple with the support of the water, which will help you to prepare for labor. If you don't swim, you can still do these exercises.

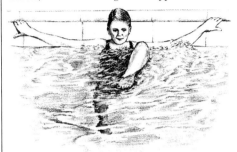 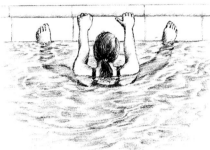

CYCLING MOVEMENTS
With your back to the rail, hold onto it with your arms stretched out straight. Raise your legs and make slow, exaggerated movements with your legs in the water. Keep cycling for a couple of minutes but don't become fatigued.

BODY MOVEMENTS
Facing the rail, put your feet flat against the side of the pool with your knees bent. Move your body from side to side. Stretch your legs out until they are straight out to either side, feet still flat against the side, and repeat the swaying movement.

Traveling

WHETHER SHORT OR LONG distance, traveling is unlikely to do you any harm during pregnancy, but do use your common sense. Don't risk getting tired with long, unbroken journeys, particularly on your own. Resist rough and jolting cross-country trips. Don't take travel sickness medication. Towards the end, try to stay close to home, within easy reach of your doctor.

DRIVING

You can drive until your size makes it hard to look over your shoulder, or until the wheel jams into your bump. For many women this occurs around month seven, for others there are no problems. It's illegal to stop wearing your seat belt just because you are pregnant. Some women lose their ability to make quick responses and to concentrate without a break. If you notice this happening, it is unwise to drive for any distance. If you suffer backache, make sure you have a proper support. Get out of the car at least every 100 miles (160 kilometers) and walk around to rest your joints and keep the circulation going.

TRAINS

Going by train is probably the most relaxing way to travel in pregnancy because there is always a toilet close by.

FLYING

Flying through time zones may be more tiring during pregnancy because of your tendency to suffer fatigue. It's all right to fly short-haul up to about 36 weeks, though for long-haul flights it's not advisable after 32 weeks. Check with your doctor and the airline first. When traveling, always fasten your seatbelt below your abdomen.

10

Looking good

In pregnancy, most women find that their skin improves and the legendary bloom appears as more blood flows under the skin, making them feel well and attractive. Exercise and a healthy diet, coupled with an awareness of the physical changes that occur in pregnancy, will contribute to your feeling happy with your changing shape and to giving you a good self-image. Taking care of your clothes, makeup and personal hygiene can also do a lot to boost morale. If you feel good, then you will probably look good too. You don't have to wear shapeless clothes; adapt your existing wardrobe for the first two trimesters.

What you wear

THE INCREASE IN THE CIRCULATION of blood throughout your body will cause you to sweat more and your vaginal secretions will also increase (see p. 154). It is therefore advisable to bathe daily (but never to douche) and to wear, whenever possible, lightweight natural fibers which won't irritate your skin or cause you to feel hot and restricted. Even in cold weather you will be astonished at how warm you feel, so wear fewer and lighter clothes than usual for your own comfort.

Being pregnant is nothing to be ashamed of, and fashion designers have increasingly been producing maternity clothes that accentuate your bump attractively, using fashionable colors and flattering and comfortable fabrics. These can be worn right through your pregnancy to the birth, and beyond. Bear in mind, however, that your bust size will increase so figure-hugging tops may no longer fit comfortably. Also, avoid any garments

that have a tight waistband or belt or fit closely around the thighs or crotch. Most women find that up to the fifth or sixth month they can get away with wearing their ordinary clothes, sometimes with a safety pin or a piece of velcro to help the waistbands meet. Any garments with a drawstring or an elasticated waist can be adapted as your abdomen swells.

It's a wonderful boost to your morale to invest in one or two really smart or glamorous outfits. So that you have several months to enjoy them, don't wait until your pregnancy is too advanced before going out shopping. Remember that you don't have to buy maternity clothes. From the standard dress racks you should be able to find fashionable clothes to wear.

TAKE PRIDE IN YOUR APPEARANCE
Your pregnant shape is something to be proud of and for you to enjoy. See your swelling body as something beautiful, and don't ever worry about it.

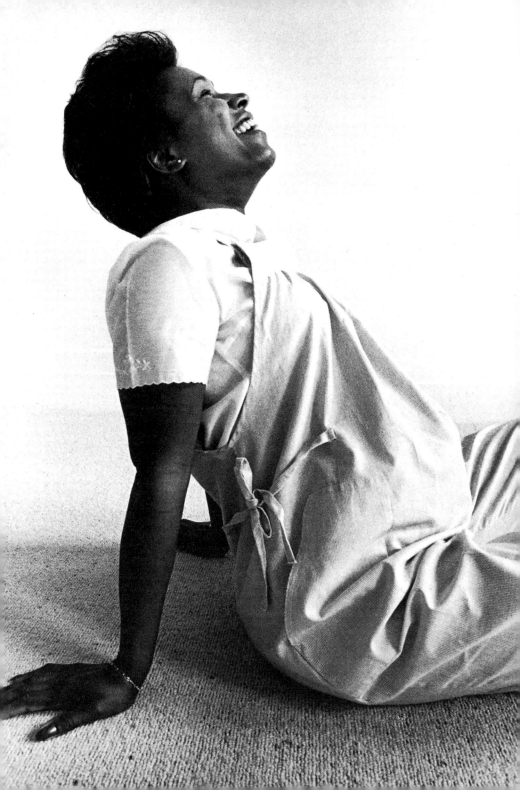

GATHERING YOUR WARDROBE

• Comfort is the watchword in pregnancy. Try to stay one step ahead of your growing size by buying clothes that are slightly too big so that you always have something to wear.

• Look in the racks of maternity clothes for ideas and make a note of the way they allow for expansion with elasticated inserts and Velcro strips, for example. You can use the same techniques to adapt your existing wardrobe.

• Front hems on maternity dresses tend to be 1 in. (2.5 cm) longer than usual, so if you make your own or buy a nonmaternity dress, check that you have the extra fabric in the hem.

• See if there is anything in your partner's wardrobe that you might borrow, for example a sweater or a shirt.

• Replace elastic in a waistband with a drawstring.

• Loose-fitting jackets, shawls, fleeces and A-line coats are the best cover-ups.

• Choose natural fabrics such as cotton, wool or silk, which are much more comfortable than synthetics, particularly in hot weather.

• Wear layers for comfort—a long shirt over a T-shirt, for example—so that if you get too hot you can easily remove the top layer.

• Big prints and wide stripes tend to make you look larger, whereas plain colors are more subtle.

• Stretch fabrics are comfortable, but avoid clingy materials.

• For a special occasion or if you need to look smart for work, look for drop-waisted dresses or suits with long-line jackets.

• To cut the cost when buying a special outfit, visit shops that specialize in nearly new maternity clothes.

• On the beach wear a muu-muu or sarong, or just a large T-shirt. Maternity swimwear is now readily available in department stores, and is generally both comfortable and stylish.

• A layered skirt with an elasticated or drawstring waistline can be worn under the armpits as a sundress, then pulled down and worn with a pretty top to make a versatile summer outfit.

A cotton tunic jumper worn over a big T-shirt is comfortable and stylish

CLOTHES FOR PREGNANCY

You don't need to buy a whole new wardrobe. A few special items supplemented with borrowed clothes will see you through.

A pair of maternity leggings with an expandable front panel will last you right through pregnancy

Footwear

Whenever you can, go barefoot. Cotton or wool socks are often the most comfortable footwear, but tights are fine provided that they are large and stretchy enough, do not have a tight waistband, and the feet leave enough room for your toes to move freely. If you can tolerate wearing the waistband under the bump, ordinary tights will be comfortable throughout pregnancy but during the third trimester you may need special maternity tights. Don't wear garters, stockings, or knee-high socks with elastic tops because these tend to make the blood stagnate in your legs.

Your feet and back are going to take quite a strain as you get heavier and your ligaments will soften and stretch. So, for the sake of foot comfort and posture, take care when choosing shoes. It is best to avoid high heels altogether as it is difficult to stand and walk well in them. In addition they can make you unstable.

Most of the time, at least, wear low-heeled shoes that are soft and comfortable. If your feet swell, tight shoes may cut into your feet, but loose-fitting shoes can cause you to slip. Therefore, for casual wear, sneakers are excellent, though the laces may be difficult to tie later in pregnancy. For summer, wear adjustable sports sandals or canvas shoes that give without pinching and allow your feet to swell freely.

Bras

You should always wear a bra in pregnancy because your breasts are becoming progressively larger and heavier, putting a strain on the supporting, nonelastic tissues. If you don't lift some of the weight from these ligaments, they will stretch and your breasts will sag permanently.

From the time your breasts start to get bigger, around weeks 6–8, wear a bra with a deep enough band under the cups, wide, comfortable straps and an adjustable fastening. If necessary, buy a bigger size as your breasts enlarge. If your breasts get very heavy, you may want to wear a lightweight bra at night.

If you are planning to breastfeed, by about week 36 you should buy a front-opening bra that will allow you to feed your baby easily. Babycare shops and department stores have a wide range of styles and sizes, but if you are an unusual shape or have a narrow or wide back, see an experienced corsetier or contact one of the childbirth organizations (see p. 244). You will be wearing this bra night and day for at least six weeks (buy at least two), so it needs to feel comfortable, like a second skin. You can buy some washable or disposable breast pads now in readiness.

MEASURING UP FOR A FEEDING BRA

Take the measurement directly under your breasts for the back size and around the fullest part of your breasts for the cup size.

TYPES OF FEEDING BRA

Both the bras illustrated below give good support, even when you are feeding.

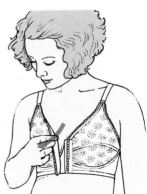

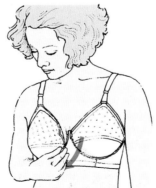

ZIP-OPENING BRA

FRONT-OPENING BRA

Skin and hair care

THERE ARE GOOD REASONS for the bloom that is said to appear on a woman's skin in pregnancy. The high level of hormones in your blood (see p. 94) affects your skin, plumping it out, giving your face a smooth, velvety appearance. Added to this, your skin acquires a rosy glow because there's more blood circulating around your body. Most women's skins improve noticeably—a dry skin becoming more supple, an oily one less shiny, and any tendency to spots disappearing—but the opposite can happen and you may have to adapt your whole beauty routine. Your face may become plumper, which tends to smooth out lines and wrinkles, making you look younger and healthier or, conversely, even chubbier than before.

You may find that your skin itches more in pregnancy, particularly over your distended stomach. Rub any kind of oil into the skin. The oil itself may not make the difference, but the massage will certainly stimulate your blood vessels and ease the irritation.

If you have put on a lot of weight, especially on your thighs, your skin may chafe. Bathe frequently, dust the area with cornstarch or talcum powder and keep it dry and cool. Wear cotton and avoid nylon tights. Calamine lotion is also soothing but the only real prevention is to cut down on your weight gain.

GENERAL SKIN CARE

- Use soap as infrequently as possible on your face and body.
- Keep hand cream and lipbalm with you to use whenever necessary.
- If you wear makeup, don't stop now; makeup is good for your skin. It slows down the water loss from the skin, helping to rehydrate it.
- Use a bath oil in your bath water. It will leave a film of lubricating oil on your skin, helping to prevent water loss.

CHLOASMA

Any areas of skin that are already pigmented, such as birthmarks, moles and freckles, can darken, especially in olive-skinned brunettes. Sunlight will intensify this so keep covered up or use a sunblock. Occasionally brown patches (chloasma or the mask of pregnancy) appear on the face and neck. They are caused by the pregnancy hormones (see p. 94) and are often noticed in women who take the contraceptive pill. Chloasma may be aggravated by a reaction to perfume, so test what you use. Don't try to bleach the marks out: cover them with a blemish stick, topped with a thin layer of foundation. They will go away within three months of delivery. Chloasma can be brought on by sunlight and it will get worse if exposed to the sun. If you can't avoid going out in the sun, use a strong sunblock. Black women may develop patches of white skin on the face and neck. These too disappear after delivery.

SPIDER VEINS

These are broken blood vessels which resemble little red spiders. They appear on the face, particularly on the cheeks. They occur when a blood vessel dilates and tiny vessels grow from this central area. They are most noticeable in fair women but will have gone within two months of delivery.

HAIR CARE

Some women notice a difference in their hair during pregnancy (see p. 101). It is a good idea to have a hairstyle that is easy to care for. You can wash your hair as often as you like, but if you notice a change in your hair, use the correct shampoo for your new hair condition. Wash your hair in the shower or use the shower attachment when you take a bath so you don't put any strain on your back.

MAKEUP CAMOUFLAGE TRICKS

If you wear makeup, a low-key, natural look is always flattering and makes the most of a fresh complexion. A style with startling details and bright colors won't do this. Pick a foundation tone a shade paler than the skin on your neck and a translucent powder. Stay away from pink blusher shades: those in the apricot range are more natural. With your eye makeup, avoid hard colors—they will compete with the sparkle in your eyes—choose soft sludgy colors instead. A natural shade of lipstick will complete the effect. There are always ways to camouflage any bad points, or at least to minimize their effects.

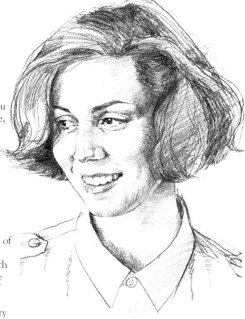

Wrinkles

If your skin becomes drier than usual, fine lines, wrinkles and crows-feet will look more obvious. Heavy foundations will accentuate them, so choose the finest texture foundation you can get, and use a fine, translucent powder.

High color

Increased blood supply can give you a permanently flushed look. To reduce this slightly, apply a matt beige foundation containing quite a lot of pigment but with no hint of pink in it. With your fingertips, stipple some onto the area of the cheeks where it's needed. Allow it to dry and then apply a thin layer of your usual foundation on top and finish with a colorless powder. This method is also good for concealing spider veins or any other red veins on the cheeks that become prominent.

Extra-greasy skin

For greasy patches of skin, use a water-based moisturizer and oil-free foundation with translucent powder.

Extra-dry skin

To deal with dry patches of skin, first apply a thin lotion that's absorbed by the skin within seconds, and on top apply a thicker kind that acts as a barrier to water loss. Covering the skin with a fine layer of suitable makeup also helps to slow down water loss. However, if your face is flaking, you won't be able to camouflage it, so abandon all makeup and moisturize your skin thoroughly for a few days. Consult your doctor if the flakiness is accompanied by redness.

Puffiness

It is most noticeable under the chin but can be camouflaged by shading a little brown blusher beneath the jaw-bone and either side of the neck. Apply blusher at the temples to draw attention to your eyes.

Dark circles

Apply a thin layer of foundation. When dry, stipple over the dark areas with an under-eye cover-up cream. Leave for a couple of minutes to set, then cover with another thin layer of foundation, blending carefully. Dust with colorless powder.

Acne

If you normally suffer from pimples or blackheads, you may find that they disappear. The fluctuation of hormones may, conversely, cause you to develop acne on the face or back for the first time. This is different from ordinary acne, so don't treat it with the usual proprietary preparations. Talk to your doctor if you are worried – it will usually have vanished by the second trimester.

To mask unsightly acne, stipple concealer or a little extra foundation over the area with your fingers. Finish with foundation and then dust with colorless powder.

Never squeeze a spot; this will spread germs into the deeper layers of the skin.

11

Rest and relaxation

During the first three months of pregnancy you are likely to feel surprisingly tired because, although your baby is still small, your body is having to cope with dramatic changes in hormone levels. By the second trimester, however, your body will have adjusted to these and it is quite common to feel full of energy rather than tired. It's in the last trimester, particularly the six weeks before your baby is born, that you once again feel quite exhausted and find that you need an additional two to four hours rest out of every 24. If it is difficult or impossible to arrange a routine break during the day, just take whatever chances you get to rest or relax. If possible, do this lying down, even if you don't go to sleep. And, any time you are sitting down, put your feet up if you can. If you ever feel extremely tired, don't try to battle on, give in.

Sleep

DURING PREGNANCY it is essential to get an adequate amount of sleep, and you should always aim for at least eight hours a night. Paradoxically, though, however tired and even exhausted you feel at times, you may find you suffer from insomnia. When I was pregnant with my first baby, I well remember sitting out the early hours of dawn wondering why my fatigue didn't let me sleep. I didn't know the reason for my wakefulness then, but theories now advanced suggest that a mother's wakefulness is due to the ever-present metabolism of her baby.

The baby is growing and developing all the time in the womb, around the clock, so its metabolism doesn't slow down when evening comes—its engine keeps running at top speed. This means that the mother's body has to constantly fuel her baby with food and oxygen, day and night, and her metabolism isn't allowed to slow down either. This is often reflected in her inability to sleep.

Don't fight sleeplessness and become resentful—it will only make your insomnia worse—and don't take any sleeping pills without consulting your doctor. If you can't get to sleep or keep waking throughout the night and become increasingly restless lying in bed, try some of the following tips:

- Take the traditional remedy of a hot, milky drink before bedtime; this helps you to relax and wind down.
- Try having a warm bath before going to bed. This soothes both mind and body, making you feel sleepy and calm as well as relaxing your muscles. For many women it acts like a knockout. Be careful, however, not to have too hot a bath before you go to bed as it may stimulate rather than relax you.
- Add aromatherapy preparations to your bath water: floral essences such as lavender, rose, geranium and chamomile are best.
- Most pregnant women seem to need to spread themselves out when they sleep. If your bed is small it might be a good idea to invest in a larger one with a good supporting mattress fairly early in your pregnancy. A larger bed will also make it easier to achieve a comfortable position, propped up with several pillows, when you come to breastfeed.
- Avoid lying on your back (see p. 146). Sleep on one side instead, in a position that you find comfortable. Get hold of some extra pillows or soft cushions and experiment with using them to make yourself more at ease. For example, when lying on your side, you might want one pillow under your bump and another between your knees and thighs (see pp. 146–147).
- Even if you have difficulty getting straight off to sleep, start going to bed earlier—you can read a good book, which will help you to relax, or do some specific relaxation exercises (see p. 143). Practice your deep breathing and concentrate on the new life inside you. Don't think of yourself as being lazy, just make sure that you get as many hours rest as you need.
- If you wake during the night, don't lie in bed fretting, get up and do something that you've been persistently putting off, or do some other useful task that could save you time the next day. Make a cup of mild herb tea, such as rosehip, chamomile or peppermint, as these may help you settle to sleep again.
- Listen to some relaxing music, either on headphones in bed, or in another room.
- Make sure you don't become too hot during the night. Remember that during pregnancy your circulation increases, which can make you feel warmer. Keep your room well ventilated with the window and door open and, if necessary, change heavy duvets or blankets for lighter bedcovers.

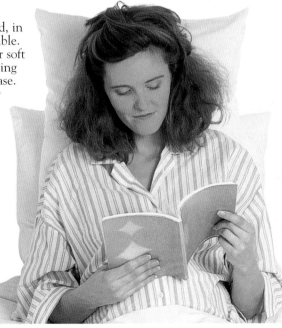

WHEN SLEEP IS DIFFICULT
Reading a good book will help you to relax. Make sure you are comfortable with your back supported by pillows.

Learning how to relax

IMPATIENCE, IRRITABILITY, an inability to concentrate and a loss of interest in sex are all signs of fatigue. Adequate rest can cure all of them. You can't always expect to get sufficient sleep at night, so you need to be alert to the possibilities of napping, or simply relaxing with your feet up, whenever the opportunity arises during the day. Long naps are not essential: five or ten minutes with your eyes closed and your feet up can be sufficiently refreshing. Something you'll never regret is learning a relaxation technique, which, once you're accustomed to using it, can recharge your batteries in a few minutes. If you want to control your body so that you can relax within 30 seconds, you might like to practice this method of instant relaxation or imagery training.

1 Arrange yourself comfortably.
2 Take a deep breath, hold for five seconds. Count to five slowly, then breathe out.
3 Tell all your muscles to relax.
4 Repeat this sequence two or three times until you're relaxed.
5 Imagine the most pleasant thought you can. A pleasant scene is ideal (see opposite). This helps you to use your imagination and to break down your mental blocks so that you can get more in touch with your body and learn to control it, which will be so useful during labor and birth.

DAYTIME REST
It is important to get enough rest, especially in the last trimester. If you find it difficult to sleep at night you should relax or have a catnap during the day.

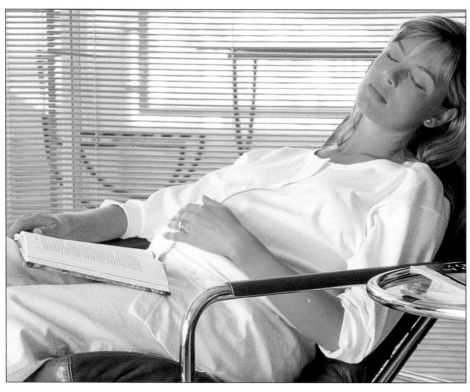

RELAXATION TECHNIQUES

PHYSICAL RELAXATION

This method involves giving orders in sequence to parts of your body to release the tension there. This is best learned through tensing and then letting go. You will feel the difference in labor, when you should be able to relax most of the muscles in your body and let the uterus contract without the rest of your body tensing. Your partner can help you by touching you where he can see you are tensing up; you can respond to his touch by letting go.

It is best to practice this drill twice a day for 15–20 minutes if you can. Practice just before meals or an hour or more after eating.

1 Find a comfortable position lying on your back or propped up with cushions.
2 Close your eyes.
3 Think about your right hand; tense it for a moment, let it go, palm upwards.
4 Tell your hand to feel heavy and warm, press your elbow into the floor or cushions, let it go.
5 Now work up through the right side of your body, through the forearm, the upper arm, into the shoulder. Raise your shoulder, let it go.
6 Repeat on the upper left side of your body. Your hands, arms and shoulders will feel heavy and warm.
7 Roll your knees outwards, relaxing your hips, and press your lower back gently into the floor or cushions. Release and let the relaxation flow into your abdomen and your chest. Tell the muscles to feel heavy and warm.
8 Your breathing should start to slow down. If it doesn't, slow it down by counting to two between each breath.
9 Now relax your neck and jaw. With your lips together, drop your jaw with your tongue on the bottom of your mouth and your cheeks loose.
10 Pay special attention to the muscles around your eyes and in your forehead; smooth away any frowns.

MENTAL RELAXATION

Once you have mastered the technique of muscle relaxation you can try relaxing your mind in this way.

1 Try clearing your mind of any stressful thoughts, anxiety or worry by breathing in and out slowly and regularly and concentrating all your attention on your breathing actions, even saying to yourself very slowly "breathe in, hold, breathe out."
2 Let pleasant thoughts flow through your head and freely associate.
3 If any worrying thought recurs, prevent it from doing so by saying "no" under your breath or return to concentrating on your deep breathing.
4 With your eyes closed, imagine a tranquil scene such as a clear, blue sky or calm, blue sea. Try to visualize something pleasant and blue because this has been found to be a particularly relaxing color.
5 Think fairly hard about your breathing and become aware of it. Feel how it is slow and natural. Concentrate on each breath as you inhale and exhale. Listen to your breathing.
6 You should be feeling calm and restful by now—it might be helpful to repeat a soothing word or mantra such as love, peace or calm, or you may prefer a word with less symbolism such as breath, earth or laugh. Think of a word or even a calming sound like "aagh" while you are breathing out.
7 Remind yourself to keep the muscles of your face, eyes and forehead relaxed and tell your forehead to feel cool.

It might help you to settle into your relaxation method if you adopt a starting routine. For example, if you repeat a mantra or drop your shoulders this can be the signal to the rest of your body to begin. Whenever you practice a relaxation method, make sure that you are breathing deeply, in the most controlled way (see p. 144).

Breathing techniques

PART OF YOUR TIME in prenatal classes will be spent learning how to relax and master the various breathing techniques. It's important to learn different types of breathing; you can use each one at different times during labor to help you to relax, conserve energy, control your body and pain, to calm you and stop you from being afraid. Realizing that you can exert some control over your body through breathing techniques will give you more confidence during labor. Here are three basic levels that will help you. Practice them with your partner, or whoever will be with you at the birth, so you can both learn the techniques to help you through labor.

DEEP BREATHING

When you breathe in you should feel the lowermost part of your lungs fill with air and your lower ribcage expand outwards and upwards. Drop your shoulders. If someone places their hands on your lower back, you should be able to move their hands with your inhalation. It feels like the end of a sigh and is followed by a slow, deep exhalation. This produces a calming influence and is ideal for the beginning and end of contractions.

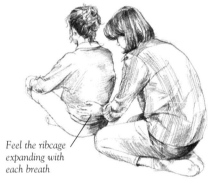

Feel the ribcage expanding with each breath

LIGHT BREATHING

Aerate only the upper part of your lungs so that the top part of your chest and your shoulder blades lift and expand. Your partner can feel this if she places her hands on your shoulder blades. Your breaths should be fast and short with your lips slightly apart. Draw the breath in through your throat. After 10 or so light breaths you may need to take a deep breath—do so. This level of breathing is useful when used in labor at the height of a contraction.

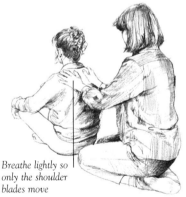

Breathe lightly so only the shoulder blades move

FEATHERLIGHT BREATHING

The method I found most useful was panting. This is taking shallow breaths and resembles what you see and hear when a dog pants. Think of this as "pant, pant, blow." One of the times when you will be asked to pant is during transition to stop you from bearing down before the cervix is fully dilated (see p. 181). When you're taking short, rapid, shallow breaths, the diaphragm is contracting and relaxing quickly and this prevents you from making a downward, concerted push. It's also useful to pant right through a painful contraction as you won't feel out of breath at the end. To stop yourself overbreathing, or hyperventilating, pant 10–15 times and then hold your breath for a count of five.

MASSAGE

Physical contact is a source of comfort and solace at any time, but especially during pregnancy. Massage can be used as a means of relaxing you, and it also brings you and your partner close together. It's very useful during the first stages of labor, not only for relieving back pain but also for helping to reassure and soothe you.

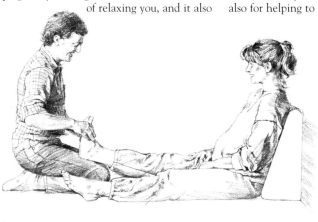

FOOT MASSAGE
With your partner well supported and comfortable, press with your thumbs on the soles and out to the edges of her feet. Firmness prevents you tickling her. Work from the heel up to the toes.

STROKING HER BROW
With your partner propped up against your chest, gently close her eyes and use your fingertips in a smooth outward movement, running your fingers out over her hair.

RELIEVE BACK PAIN
With your partner lying on her side, feel for the base of the tail bone between the buttocks and press firmly with the heel of your hand. Make small circular movements to relieve back pain. Now move your hands down to her knees and smooth her thighs up to her buttocks.

Comfortable positions

AS YOUR ABDOMEN gets larger, sitting or lying in your usual positions can become uncomfortable. If you lie flat on your back for any length of time, especially in later pregnancy, the baby's weight presses down on major blood vessels running up your

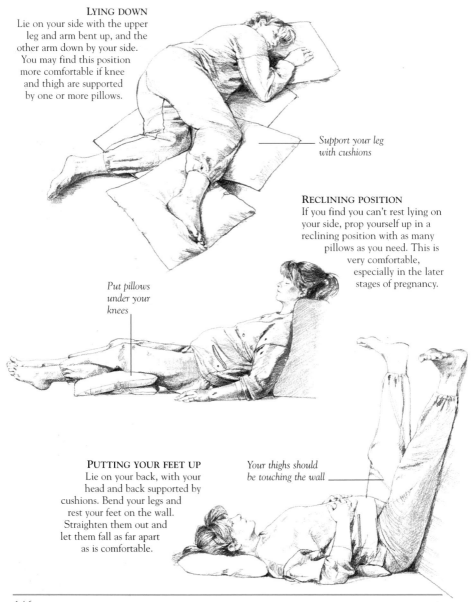

LYING DOWN
Lie on your side with the upper leg and arm bent up, and the other arm down by your side. You may find this position more comfortable if knee and thigh are supported by one or more pillows.

Support your leg with cushions

RECLINING POSITION
If you find you can't rest lying on your side, prop yourself up in a reclining position with as many pillows as you need. This is very comfortable, especially in the later stages of pregnancy.

Put pillows under your knees

PUTTING YOUR FEET UP
Lie on your back, with your head and back supported by cushions. Bend your legs and rest your feet on the wall. Straighten them out and let them fall as far apart as is comfortable.

Your thighs should be touching the wall

back. This can make you uncomfortable and dizzy as your blood pressure drops and it can aggravate hemorrhoids. For these reasons, it's not advisable to sleep, rest or exercise on your back. Carefully arranged pillows and floor cushions help, but don't lie with too many pillows under your head or your spine will be too curved. When sitting, don't cross your legs or bend them tightly as this may aggravate varicose veins. Try the positions below and always be aware of maintaining good posture.

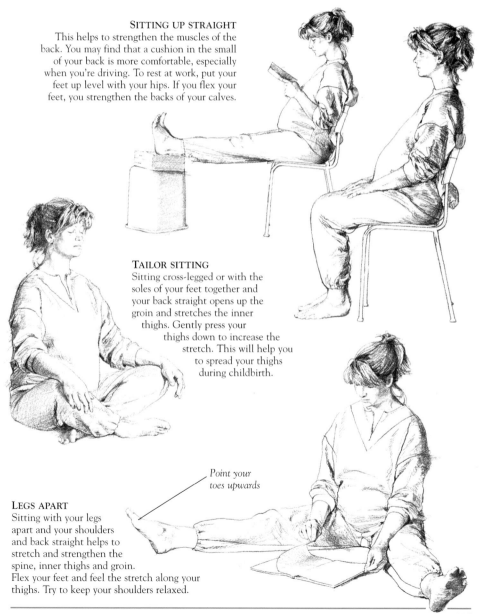

SITTING UP STRAIGHT
This helps to strengthen the muscles of the back. You may find that a cushion in the small of your back is more comfortable, especially when you're driving. To rest at work, put your feet up level with your hips. If you flex your feet, you strengthen the backs of your calves.

TAILOR SITTING
Sitting cross-legged or with the soles of your feet together and your back straight opens up the groin and stretches the inner thighs. Gently press your thighs down to increase the stretch. This will help you to spread your thighs during childbirth.

Point your toes upwards

LEGS APART
Sitting with your legs apart and your shoulders and back straight helps to stretch and strengthen the spine, inner thighs and groin. Flex your feet and feel the stretch along your thighs. Try to keep your shoulders relaxed.

12
Common complaints

COMPLAINT	CAUSES
ABDOMINAL PAIN 2nd & 3rd trimester	Round ligament pain occurs during pregnancy when the ligaments supporting the uterus stretch.
BACKACHE 1st, 2nd & 3rd trimester	Progesterone causes softening and stretching of the ligaments, most importantly in the pelvic joints. The ligaments supporting the spine also relax, which puts extra strain on the muscles and joints of the lower spine, pelvis and hips. Bad posture can make backache worse.
BLEEDING GUMS 1st, 2nd & 3rd trimester	The gums thicken and soften due to the influence of the pregnancy hormones, which increases the body's blood supply. They swell, especially around the teeth, and food tends to collect in the hollows at the base of the teeth, allowing bacteria to grow and multiply, causing tooth decay and possibly gum infection (gingivitis).
CONSTIPATION 1st, 2nd & 3rd trimester	Progesterone causes relaxation of the muscles of the intestine and thus slows down bowel movements. Bowel contents tend to stagnate and dry out so that the stools become hard and painful to pass.
CRAMPS 3rd trimester	Thought to be a result of low levels of calcium in the blood. In rare cases it is due to a lack of salt in the diet.
CRAVINGS 1st, 2nd & 3rd trimester	Thought to be related to high levels of progesterone.
DISCOMFORT IN BED 3rd trimester	As a result of indigestion or heartburn (see p. 150) or, when you lie down, the enlarging uterus presses on the diaphragm, the stomach and the ribcage.

Ailments in pregnancy

PREGNANCY IS NOT AN ILLNESS and most women have normal, healthy pregnancies that proceed without any problems. However, there is no denying that pregnancy can be an uncomfortable time. Many of the common complaints of pregnancy are irritating rather than real cause for concern, and being prepared for them is half the battle. Many of the aches and pains of pregnancy are due to a combination of tiredness and carrying around that extra weight. However, if you are at all worried about anything, don't be afraid to consult your doctor or midwife. He or she will be happy to discuss any anxieties that you have and will be pleased to be able to reassure you that all is well.

SYMPTOMS	TREATMENTS
Either felt as stabbing, cramplike pain when you get up after sitting or lying for a time or a dragging pain on one side only.	None. Pain normally spasmodic so painkillers are not worthwhile. Apply a hot water bottle to relax muscles.
General ache across the lower back. Sacroiliac pain is classically across the top of the buttocks and extending down into them.	Good posture and exercises to strengthen the spine (see p. 128) to make it more supple. Avoid very high heels; wear sensible shoes with a moderate heel. Have a good firm mattress on your bed. Avoid heavy lifting (see p. 121). If the pain runs down your leg towards the foot, consult your doctor in case of a slipped disc. Try to avoid analgesics. Massage (see p. 145) may help.
Gums are tender and bleed after brushing or eating hard foods. Gingivitis causes more bleeding than is normal after brushing.	Attention to oral hygiene is essential, with regular brushing of the teeth after food. Visit your dentist regularly but tell him you are pregnant as you should avoid X-rays at this time. There is no truth in the tale that the baby takes calcium from your teeth. Gingivitis should be reported at once to your dentist.
Infrequent hard stools. Pain in the lower abdomen.	Obey the call to empty your bowels whenever your body tells you. Take plenty of dietary fiber and lots of fluid, preferably water. Regular exercise helps too. Avoid strong laxatives.
Pain in the leg and foot, sufficiently painful to wake you. A hard knot of pain often followed for some hours by a general ache.	Very firm massage, possibly for several minutes; it also helps to flex the foot up and push into the heel (see p. 127). If cramping persists, see your doctor, who may prescribe calcium tablets.
Strong desire for certain foods which prevents sleep and relaxation.	Indulge yourself provided the foods aren't fattening.
Shortness of breath, acid regurgitation, soreness and tenderness of the ribs.	Try sitting up in bed with two or three extra pillows or try some of the positions on p. 146. Get a firm bed and avoid heartburn (see p. 150).

COMPLAINT	CAUSES
FAINTING 1st & 3rd trimester	Pooling of the blood in the legs and feet when standing, together with the demands of the uterus for an increased blood supply, causes the brain to be relatively deprived of blood.
FLATULENCE 1st & 3rd trimester	Unwittingly swallowing air; also eating certain foods, e.g., pulses, fried foods and onions. In pregnancy the intestine is more sluggish and the wind may be more difficult to expel.
FREQUENT URINATION 1st & 3rd trimester	Early in pregnancy hormonal changes lead to differences in muscle tone that affect the bladder; also the growing uterus presses on the bladder, causing it to empty itself more frequently. Later in pregnancy the weight of the uterus on the bladder reduces its capacity.
HEMORRHOIDS (PILES) 2nd & 3rd trimester	The pressure of the baby's head in the pelvis in late pregnancy may obstruct the blood vessels in the rectum, impairing the return of blood from the pelvic organs and causing ballooning of the veins around the rectum. Anything that increases pressure in the abdomen, such as constipation, chronic coughing and lifting, will worsen hemorrhoids.
HEARTBURN 3rd trimester	The valve at the entrance to your stomach relaxes in pregnancy, allowing small amounts of acid to get into the esophagus (the tube running from your mouth to your stomach).
INCONTINENCE 3rd trimester	Pressure of the enlarging uterus on the bladder, thus reducing its capacity, and the inability of the pelvic floor muscles to stop leakage when you cough or laugh.
INSOMNIA 1st, 2nd & 3rd trimester	The general increase in your metabolism. The baby's metabolism doesn't distinguish between day and night so it may kick you at night. Also sweating and frequent urination may cause you to wake.
ITCHING 2nd & 3rd trimester	Itching is common and is caused by increased blood supply to the skin. If the itching becomes troublesome or generalized, particularly in the latter stages of pregnancy, it could be a potentially dangerous liver disorder, obstetric cholestasis.
MORNING SICKNESS 1st trimester	Sudden high levels of hormones, particularly human chorionic gonadotrophin (HCG), the production of which closely parallels the time of nausea. It is not clear, though, why it affects some women and not others. Diet before conception can predispose to nausea in early pregnancy, particularly a diet low in vitamins, minerals and carbohydrates. Tiredness also contributes, making nausea more severe, though it is not a direct cause.

SYMPTOMS	TREATMENTS
Dizziness, spinning, unsteadiness and need to sit or lie down.	Avoid standing still for long periods of time. Don't jump up from sitting too suddenly. Take care when getting out of a hot bath. Keep yourself as cool as possible in hot weather. If you feel faintness coming on, lie down with your head flat and if possible raise your legs slightly.
Distension of the intestine, rumbling of the stomach, frequent passing of gas.	Try not to gulp air and avoid problem foods. Peppermint and hot drinks may help.
Urgent need to pass urine, even the smallest amounts, and at frequent intervals day and night.	Nothing much you can do except reduce your liquid intake before going to bed. Later in pregnancy, try rocking backwards and forwards as you pass urine. This lessens pressure on the bladder and it may be more completely emptied. If you have any pain or blood when passing urine, see your doctor.
Itching, soreness, severe pain when passing stools, slight blood loss if the hemorrhoid is large and prolapses outside the rectum.	Prevent hemorrhoids with a diet high in roughage, plenty of fluids and exercise, thus avoiding constipation. Try not to strain when you move your bowels. Minor hemorrhoids will get better after delivery but if they persist you may need soothing creams. Keep the anal area clean to avoid irritation. If hemorrhoids itch badly, apply an ice pack or crushed ice in a plastic bag.
Burning sensation behind the breastbone sometimes accompanied by the regurgitation of sour fluid.	Avoid the foods which give you trouble and don't eat a meal just before going to bed. Prop yourself up in bed and try a warm milk drink. Antacid medicines (see p. 114) may be prescribed.
Leakage of urine whenever you increase pressure within the abdomen, e.g., bending down, laughing.	Empty your bladder often, avoid heavy lifting and constipation. Do your pelvic floor exercise regularly (see p. 125).
Difficulty going to sleep, or getting back to sleep after waking.	Wear light night clothes to avoid overheating. A hot milk drink or a hot bath (see pp. 140–141) before bed may help. Try a good book. Rarely will doctors prescribe sleeping pills except in the last trimester if the problem is leading to exhaustion.
Obstetric cholestasis causes generalized itching of the skin. Other symptoms may include dark urine, pale stools, jaundice.	Close monitoring under consultant care is essential. This may involve regular scans, cardiographs, blood tests and placental blood flow scans. Whatever treatment is given, early delivery is thought to be vital, with delivery considered desirable by 37–38 weeks.
Feelings of nausea at the sight or smell of food, or the smell of cigarette smoke. Occasionally accompanied by vomiting.	Eat little and often and avoid foods that make you nauseous. Don't get overtired, this will make your nausea worse. If you understand why you are feeling ill, you may be more relaxed about it. Try the diet ideas (see p. 116), suck peppermints or nibble dried fruits or dried biscuits; keep up your fluid intake. Talk to other women; if you know you're not the only one it may help. Your doctor will be loath to prescribe anything for you.

COMPLAINT	CAUSES
NASAL DISCOMFORT 1st, 2nd & 3rd trimester	Softening and thickening of the mucous membranes in the nose. Increase in blood supply to the lining of the nose due to high levels of pregnancy hormones. You may wake with a blocked nose in the morning. Rough blowing may rupture tiny blood vessels.
EDEMA 3rd trimester	Increase in fluid retained by your body and stagnation of this fluid in the lower parts of your body and your fingers. Pressure of the uterus on the blood vessels that return blood to the heart from the lower parts of the body. Can be associated with pre-eclampsia (see p. 162).
PELVIC DISCOMFORT 3rd trimester	The baby's head presses upon nerves, causing pain in the groin, particularly when the head is engaged in the pelvic cavity at the end of pregnancy.
PIGMENTATION 2nd & 3rd trimester	Increased production of melanocyte stimulating hormone (see p. 94). Made worse by exposure to strong sunlight.
RASHES 3rd trimester	Excess weight gain, poor hygiene and sweating in the folds of the skin.
RIB PAIN 3rd trimester	Costal margin pain results from the compression of the ribs as the uterus rises, the high position of the baby's head and excessive kicking by the baby.
SHORTNESS OF BREATH 3rd trimester	Pressure on the diaphragm prevents easy breathing. Lying down can also push the uterus and baby up against the diaphragm.
STRETCHMARKS 2nd & 3rd trimester	Depends on your skin type, and its elasticity. However, whatever your skin type, excess weight gain may cause stretchmarks (see p. 100).
SWEATING 2nd & 3rd trimester	Increased blood supply causes the blood vessels beneath the skin to dilate (see p. 98).

SYMPTOMS	TREATMENTS
Stuffiness in the nose, unexpected nosebleeds, congestion upon waking or runny nose.	Treat your nose gently. Avoid dry dusty atmospheres. Don't use a nasal spray without talking to your doctor. If you have a nosebleed, apply gentle pressure to the bridge of your nose. Lean forward slightly.
Swelling of the hands and ankles. Shoes feel tight. Your fingers may feel stiff in the morning.	Avoid standing, particularly in hot weather. Rest with your legs up, and rest at least once during the day. Avoid very salty foods. If you have severe edema, your doctor may restrict your salt intake and use diuretics to get rid of excess fluid.
Pain in the groin and down the inside of the thighs, particularly bad after walking or exercising. Pins and needles spreading down the back of your legs.	Rest, avoid violent exercise and take an analgesic such as paracetamol, but consult your doctor first.
Darkening around the nipple and areola, down the center of the abdomen (linea nigra), deepening of pigmentation in freckles or birthmarks, mask across the face (butterfly mask) and down the sides (chloasma).	Use sunblock when you are out in strong sunshine. Don't ever bleach the skin. The pigmentation will fade within a few months of delivery.
Intertrigo is a red skin rash occurring where heavy folds of skin become irritated by sweat. Usually occurs under heavy breasts or in the groin area.	Keep the areas clean and apply a soothing lotion such as calamine. Dust with talcum powder after bathing or showering to make sure it is dry.
Soreness and tenderness, usually on the right side. The pain is felt just below the breasts. It is severe when sitting up straight.	The pain will disappear as soon as the baby's head drops into the pelvic cavity prior to birth (or earlier in some women, especially those pregnant with their first child). Try not to compress the ribs: either sit up straight or lie down.
Shortness of breath on exertion.	Try to be less active. Rest in the day and go to bed early. If breathlessness is accompanied by chest pain or swelling, consult your doctor.
Silver marks on the skin of the thighs, abdomen and breasts.	Creams and ointments will have no effect. Eventually the marks will become smaller, narrower and a light silver color, but they rarely disappear altogether. Make sure you do not put on too much weight too quickly.
Intense perspiration after light exertion or on waking at night.	Wear light cotton clothing and cotton underwear. Drink more to replace lost fluids.

COMPLAINT	CAUSES
TASTE DISTURBANCES 1st, 2nd & 3rd trimester	Thought to be related to the pregnancy hormones.
THRUSH 1st, 2nd & 3rd trimester	The yeast candida albicans infects the vagina. Why it is more common in pregnancy is not known. The yeast can infect the baby's mouth at birth.
TIREDNESS 1st, 2nd & 3rd trimester	Sometimes because of worry, lack of sleep (see insomnia), poor nutrition, and towards the end of pregnancy the sheer burden of carrying around the unborn baby. Your body has to support both you and your baby.
URINARY TRACT INFECTION (CYSTITIS) 1st, 2nd & 3rd trimester	Slackening and relaxation of the muscle wall predisposes the bladder to infection at any time during pregnancy. The high level of progesterone is the cause. Symptoms may appear gradually over several weeks or months.
VAGINAL DISCHARGE 1st, 2nd & 3rd trimester	Increased blood supply and softening and thickening of the mucous membranes result in a normal increase of mucoid discharge. Brown or yellow discharge could be cervical erosion, when increased secretions may cause an ulcer in the upper vagina. This ulcer could be damaged during sexual intercourse and spots of blood, not of a continuous nature, may appear. Heavy or smelly discharge may be a symptom of a sexually transmitted disease (STD).
VARICOSE VEINS 1st, 2nd & 3rd trimester	A family history of varicose veins may mean that you develop them too. Near to term the baby's head can press down on the pelvic veins, causing blood to pool in the veins of the legs, and the result is ballooning of these veins. Standing for long periods of time will make swollen veins worse. Sitting with tightly crossed legs cuts off blood flow. Excess weight gain also causes the veins to dilate. Varicose veins on the vulva may result if the baby's head is interfering with the flow of blood there. The vulva then becomes swollen and congested.
VISUAL DISTURBANCES 1st, 2nd & 3rd trimester	Retention of fluid. If contact lenses feel different, this is because the eyeball has slightly changed shape with the increase in fluid.

SYMPTOMS	TREATMENTS
Often a metallic taste. Appreciation of the taste of certain foods alters. Coffee, alcohol and spicy foods, for example, become less palatable than before. Often increased liking for sugar and sweet things.	None.
Thick, white curdy discharge accompanied by intense itchiness. There can be some pain when passing urine.	Antifungals in the form of a suppository and a cream will be prescribed. They clear up the infection in two to three days. If the baby contracts the infection at delivery, a course of medicine will quickly clear it up. Try not to wear tight underpants.
Strong desire to sleep at odd times and needing more sleep at night. Legs ache and seem unable to carry you any further later in pregnancy.	Avoid overactivity. Sleep or rest whenever you can. Eat nutritious foods little and often to keep up your energy. Go to bed early. Get others to do the work.
Increased desire to pass urine accompanied by discomfort and pain. Urine may contain spots of blood. Dull discomfort in the lower abdomen.	Try to drink plenty of water. See your doctor. Your urine will be tested and you will be given specific anti-infectives to eradicate the infection.
Slight increase over normal of the clear, white discharge which does not cause soreness, pain or irritation. Discolored or smelly discharge.	If the discharge is simply increased mucus, don't worry. Don't douche or use a vaginal deodorant. Wear cotton underwear and change it frequently, especially in warm weather. If the discharge is discolored, smelly or includes spots of blood, inform your doctor.
Skin may be irritated or itchy at first, or there may be a dull aching pain. Then the veins start to appear as dark purplish lines on the legs. A heavy feeling in the vulva.	Avoid standing around. Wear support tights; put them on before you get up in the morning after lying with your feet raised for a few minutes. Sleep with your feet on a pillow. Do exercises to improve circulation in your legs and feet (see p. 127). For varicosity of the vulva, sleep with your bottom on a pillow or wear a sanitary pad firmly against the swollen part.
Long or short sightedness may develop. Contact lenses may be uncomfortable to wear.	If you notice anything different, go to an optician. If you wear contact lenses, tell the staff at the prenatal clinic. You may have to stop wearing them during pregnancy.

13

Special care pregnancies

Not every pregnancy is textbook but it's wrong to view some events, such as a multiple pregnancy, for example, as abnormal. You may have complications or unforeseen problems, but early intervention can help in most cases, provided the warning signs are recognized.

Anemia

PREEXISTING ANEMIA is no preclusion to pregnancy—more than 90 percent of women may be slightly anemic before they conceive. The commonest form is iron-deficiency anemia (when the hemoglobin level is less than 12.8 gm/dl blood— see p. 73) due to loss of blood at menstruation. Before you become pregnant, increase your intake of iron-rich foods and consult your doctor, who can correct iron-deficiency anemia simply with a course of iron supplements.

Prepartum hemorrhage

BEFORE 24 WEEKS, bleeding from the vagina may result in a miscarriage (see p. 160). After this time the fetus is considered viable, that is, it could survive outside its mother's womb. Any bleeding after 24 weeks is known as prepartum hemorrhage. The two main causes of this kind of bleeding derive from the placenta, and are known medically as abruptio placentae and placenta previa.

ABRUPTIO PLACENTAE

If the placenta detaches itself from the wall of the uterus it will bleed. The blood gradually builds up until it escapes around the membranes and through the cervix. Treatment may be bedrest and monitoring with ultrasound, followed by induction or possible cesarean delivery if necessary. Severe abruption is a medical emergency and will involve blood transfusions and emergency cesarean delivery.

PLACENTA PREVIA

When the placenta is attached to the lower segment of the uterine wall, it is known as placenta previa. If it lies partially or wholly over the cervix, it could be dangerous during labor as it could cause bleeding and cut off the fetal blood supply. Placenta previa is detected by ultrasound scan. If there is any bleeding, you may be admitted to hospital, or you will be closely checked by the prenatal clinic and your baby delivered by elective cesarean section.

Diabetes

MOST WOMEN who are diabetic have straightforward normal pregnancies, although their diabetes must be controlled before conception. It's essential for your health and that of the baby to keep your diabetes stable, so you'll be seen more frequently than usual at the prenatal clinic. You should pay special attention to your diet and your doctor will control your drug requirements carefully as they may vary during pregnancy. The presence of sugar in your urine (see p. 72) doesn't necessarily mean you're diabetic. Pregnancy may often cause the kidney to let sugar filter through from the blood to the urine. Special blood tests will be done to determine whether or not you do in fact have diabetes.

Ectopic pregnancy

IN AN ECTOPIC PREGNANCY, the fertilized ovum fails to reach the uterine cavity, becoming trapped instead in the fallopian tube and growing in its cavity. An ectopic pregnancy usually proceeds only to about 8–10 weeks, at which point the tube usually bursts. Before this there may be symptoms that signal all is not well, although in many cases it comes as a complete surprise. There may be pain in the lower abdomen, usually on one side, vaginal bleeding, and sometimes the woman may faint. If you have any of these symptoms you should go to your doctor. The pregnancy must be surgically removed from the fallopian tube. Sometimes it's necessary to remove the whole tube, depending on how much damage has been done. Unfortunately, it's likely that fertility is reduced after one ectopic pregnancy. Its incidence may have increased due to the use of IUDs, which can cause inflammation and subsequent blockage of the fallopian tube.

WARNING SIGNS

Contact the hospital maternity unit or your doctor immediately if you have any of the following symptoms, and while you are waiting, rest in bed. If your doctor cannot come quickly, call an ambulance and alert the clinic that you are coming into hospital:
● very severe nausea or vomiting several times within a short period, say two hours
● vaginal bleeding
● severe headache that doesn't go away, particularly in the second half of pregnancy
● a fever of 100°F (37.8°C) or over, regardless of the cause
● severe abdominal pain
● a sudden reduction in the amount of urine you pass, for example if you don't urinate for 24 hours even though you're taking in normal quantities of fluid during that time
● rupture of the membranes
● absence of fetal movement for 24 hours from the 30th week of your pregnancy onwards
● sudden swelling of the ankles, feet, fingers and face
● sudden blurring of vision.

Heart disease

WOMEN WITH PREEXISTING heart disease often have easy pregnancies and labors; some even find their condition improves. Nowadays heart disease is not considered a bar to pregnancy except for women who have serious limitations of normal life. You'll be closely supervised and you must take great care to rest so that no extra strain is put on the heart. Extra rest should include at least two naps during the day and 12 hours' sleep at night. If you get a chest infection, a raised temperature or notice swelling of the hands, face or feet, contact your doctor.

Hypertension

HYPERTENSION is the medical term for raised blood pressure. Blood pressure is given as two figures, for example 120/70 (see p. 73). Doctors are more concerned about a rise in the lower number, the diastolic pressure, which is a measure of the heart pumping when you are at rest. If you know that you have high blood pressure, you should consult your doctor before becoming pregnant. With proper prenatal care, there's no reason why you shouldn't have a normal pregnancy and labor, though you're more likely to be admitted to a hospital early. Raised blood pressure in later pregnancy can be a sign of pre-eclampsia, which is always taken seriously (see p. 162).

The difficulty with taking blood pressure readings is that anxiety and stress may mean that the problem appears worse because your reading is high as a result of your emotional state, although this generally affects only the systolic (higher) measurement. It would be wise to rest often and curtail physical exercise so that strain on the heart is minimized. If you become anxious in the clinic, practice your relaxation techniques (see p. 143).

Incompetent cervix

UNDER NORMAL CIRCUMSTANCES the cervix remains closed so that the fetus is retained in the body of the uterus and doesn't fall into the vagina. If the end of the cervical canal is open, it is described as an incompetent cervix. The most usual causes of incompetent cervix are either late (after 12 weeks) surgical termination of pregnancy or cone biopsy of the cervix, either of which may damage the muscle fibers that hold the cervix closed.

Usually an incompetent cervix remains hidden until the first miscarriage has occurred. The cervical canal starts to open by the 14th week and by the 20th has dilated to about 1 in. (2.5 cm), which is large enough for the bag of waters to bulge into the cervix and eventually break. There is usually a sudden loss of water, followed by a miscarriage with little pain.

A special stitch is inserted around the cervix to tighten it; this is known as a Shirodkar or purse-string suture. This can be performed before or during the next pregnancy. The cervix is usually stitched during pregnancy, around the 14th week, under a general anesthetic. This treatment has a high success rate and most pregnancies proceed normally. At the 36th–38th week, the stitch is removed, labor usually beginning shortly afterwards either naturally or by induction, but some women do go to term.

Multiple pregnancy

TWINS ARE EITHER IDENTICAL—formed from a single egg—or nonidentical when two eggs are fertilized. With identical twins, both babies usually share the placenta. Ultrasound will confirm the presence of twins or larger multiples from about the eighth week of pregnancy, but your doctor may be on the alert for twins anyway if:
• there are twins in your family
• your uterus is consistently bigger than your dates suggest
• two fetal hearts can be picked up with an electronic fetal stethoscope
• as pregnancy progresses, two heads can be felt as well as multiple arms and legs.

If you are carrying twins, you will have special prenatal care with an emphasis on avoiding anemia (see p. 156). Expect to have regular checks on blood pressure to make sure it doesn't rise, and take plenty of rest to keep your blood pressure low and damp down the sensitivity of the uterus so that it doesn't go into labor prematurely. A multiple pregnancy puts extra pressure on your joints and ligaments and on your digestive organs. Attend promptly to any

TWIN PRESENTATIONS

The most common presentation for twins is for both to be in the cephalic position (below left) so delivery is usually straightforward. If one is breech and the other cephalic (below right), the cephalic baby is usually born first, stretching the birth canal so that the second baby can be delivered easily. If both babies are breech, if one baby is lying transversely, that is across the womb, or if the babies are large, a cesarean section may be performed.

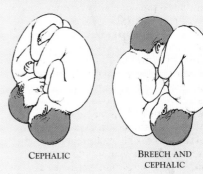

CEPHALIC   BREECH AND CEPHALIC

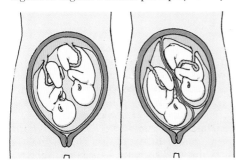

IDENTICAL TWINS
Developing from the fertilization of one egg that splits into separate cells, identical twins are always the same sex and look alike. They usually share a placenta but have their own cord and sac.

NON-IDENTICAL TWINS
The result of two eggs that have been fertilized by two sperm, non-identical twins each have their own placenta and need be no more alike than any two children in the same family.

irritating minor symptoms such as flatulence and dyspepsia. Because the uterus may crowd out your digestive organs, eat little and often. Salads and light nutritious snacks will prevent you becoming too uncomfortable. If you take care not to gain too much weight and pay particular attention to posture, most complications can be avoided.

The large size of the uterus can also cause shortness of breath, piles, varicose veins and abdominal discomfort. At the first sign of any of these symptoms, alert your doctor and you'll be given help, advice and treatment. You may suffer from more nausea in the first trimester but this is by no means the rule. You will probably have to have your babies in a hospital because of the risk to the second baby if it isn't born immediately after the first.

MISCARRIAGE

Sometimes known as spontaneous abortion, miscarriage is when the embryo or fetus is expelled from the uterus before the 24th week of pregnancy. After the 24th week, if the baby does not survive, it is called a stillbirth (see p. 212).

Doctors use the words abortion and miscarriage synonymously, and medically speaking there is absolutely no difference. To most people, however, the word "abortion" is usually associated with the medical termination of pregnancy, whereas a miscarriage is always something that occurs spontaneously.

Overall the frequency of miscarriage may be as high as one in ten pregnancies and it is first pregnancies that are more likely to miscarry—about one-third of all first pregnancies abort. This is thought to happen for two reasons. First, a young uterus may need to mature by having a "trial run" before it is ready to carry a pregnancy to full term. Second, it is thought that the majority of these miscarriages are due to a defect in either the sperm or the ovum, resulting in an abnormal embryo, which the body then rejects.

The majority of miscarriages, however, occur during the first trimester, and most of these pregnancies would never have developed properly, revealing a deformity in the baby or a placenta that has failed to develop adequately. Indeed, many miscarriages occur before the woman is even aware that she is pregnant.

Miscarriages, especially those that occur after the first trimester, can also be caused by the following conditions:
● an incompetent cervix—for various reasons the cervix sometimes fails to remain closed (see p. 158)
● an incompatible blood type (see p. 162) which causes antibodies to your partner's blood type to develop, resulting in the death of the fetus
● placental insufficiency—if the placenta is not functioning well or has not developed properly, it will not be able to nourish the baby adequately
● diabetes.

IF A MISCARRIAGE THREATENS
● Call or visit your doctor.
● If you pass any clots or membranes, or the fetus and the placenta, collect them in a clean container and keep for the doctor to examine.
● Don't take any medicines or alcohol.
● Lie flat if the bleeding seems heavy and keep your room cool.

What happens
Miscarriage is nearly always heralded by bleeding from the vagina, with or without abdominal pain. An early miscarriage may cause no more discomfort than a menstrual period without menstrual cramps. In some instances vaginal bleeding does not mean that a miscarriage will inevitably occur, but there's no way of you knowing, so you should always consult your doctor.

As far as a doctor is concerned, any bleeding during the first 24 weeks of pregnancy is considered to be a threatened abortion until proved otherwise. The bleeding may be light or heavy, accompanied by the passage of mucus or not; there may be a small amount of backache and discomfort in the lower part of the abdomen. Doctors have come up with no better cause for a threatened abortion in the early stages of pregnancy than "hormone imbalance" or a "hormone insufficiency" which doesn't suppress the next period. If bleeding of this type occurs and the hormone levels remain low then abortion will almost certainly follow.

There is no specific treatment for a threatened miscarriage. Doctors used to suggest complete bedrest, but this does not make any difference to the eventual outcome; unfortunately, if a miscarriage is going to occur, it will happen whether you rest or not. If, however, the bleeding stops and the pregnancy continues normally, you might be advised to refrain from penetrative sexual intercourse and strenuous exercise until fetal movements have been felt, which happens at about 20 weeks with a first baby and 18 weeks with second and subsequent babies.

TYPES OF MISCARRIAGE

Threatened abortion An abortion is possible but not inevitable; there is bleeding from the vagina, rarely accompanied by pain.

Inevitable abortion Vaginal bleeding is accompanied by pain due to the uterus contracting. If on internal examination the cervix is dilated, an abortion is bound to occur.

Missed abortion The fetus is no longer alive but is still in the uterus. The fetus will be expelled by the uterus eventually.

Complete abortion The fetus and placenta have been expelled from the uterus.

Incomplete abortion The fetus has been lost but some of the products of conception are still in the uterus and will have to be removed surgically.

Recurrent abortion An abortion has occurred on more than one occasion, for different reasons and at different stages of the pregnancy.

Habitual abortion Three or more miscarriages have occurred at the same time and possibly for the same reason in each pregnancy. High temperature and abdominal pain following the abortion indicate infection.

Inevitable abortion

If the bleeding does not stop, and if abdominal pain appears or worsens, which usually means that the uterus is contracting to expel the fetus, most medical experts agree that efforts should not be made to try to salvage the pregnancy.

If the abortion is incomplete, you will need surgical attention. Examination of the products of conception doesn't always reveal that part has been left behind in the uterus, but this becomes obvious when bleeding persists after the miscarriage has taken place. However, it's important to have the uterus cleaned out to avoid further hemorrhage and pelvic infection. This involves admission to a hospital for one day for an D&C (dilation and curettage) under a general anesthetic. During this operation any abnormal material is removed from the uterus.

Emotional effects

Miscarriage at any time, but particularly one that occurs during the second trimester of pregnancy, has a profound psychological effect on a woman. This is due not only to the loss of the baby and the wide range of emotions resulting from that, but also because of the sudden withdrawal of pregnancy hormones without the reward of having a baby.

There are many fears—about your own inadequacy, that you may never be able to carry another baby, that your fertility may be permanently affected, that you had an abnormal baby this time and that you could have another next time.

I also think that there is a feeling of real bereavement. I suffered a miscarriage myself at 14 weeks and was actually shown the fetus, which was well enough formed to distinguish that it was a boy. For about six weeks afterwards I found myself in a deeply depressed, depersonalized state, unwilling to communicate with other people or participate in day-to-day activities.

After a miscarriage your emotions need careful handling, because they may be complicated by feelings of guilt and blame that could trigger depression or drive a wedge between you and your partner. Try to talk about your feelings to each other and with your doctor.

The next pregnancy

When you start the next pregnancy, of course, is a matter of choice and planning and you should take as much time as you need. From a medical point of view, sexual relations can begin as soon as the bleeding has stopped, and my advice has always been to try to forget the first mishap and to start a second pregnancy as soon as you both want to.

Pre-eclampsia

ALSO KNOWN AS pre-eclamptic toxemia (PET), pre-eclampsia is a potentially serious condition that can affect as many as one in ten women, especially first-time mothers and women carrying more than one baby. It's unique to pregnancy, starting at any time in the second half. It's not known precisely what causes the condition, but it does tend to run in families. It is also known that it arises in the placenta so the baby may grow more slowly than normal.

The pregnancy cannot be restored to normal once you have pre-eclampsia, so your condition and that of your baby will be monitored closely, probably in a hospital or possibly in a special day unit. In this way delivery can be arranged quickly before serious complications arise. For almost every mother, delivery of her baby reverses the condition, although your blood pressure may remain raised for up to six weeks after the birth, requiring treatment to bring it under control. If your pre-eclampsia was so severe that you

SIGNS OF PRE-ECLAMPSIA

Pre-eclampsia does not have any outward symptoms, and many women who are diagnosed as having it are surprised and frustrated, as they may feel perfectly well in themselves. Staff at prenatal checks will be alerted to its presence if:
● you have raised blood pressure, especially if it is consistently raised over a couple of weeks. An increase that would ordinarily be insignificant may be considered abnormal during pregnancy
● protein is detected in your urine—it signals potential damage to the kidneys
● there is swelling (edema) to the feet, ankles or hands; it can also affect the face, causing puffiness to the neck and eyes
● you suddenly gain weight excessively.

were in danger of convulsions, leaving the hospital early isn't recommended as the risk of having a fit remains for up to five days after the birth.

Rhesus incompatibility

THE BLOOD SAMPLE taken at your first prenatal visit reveals your blood group, (see p. 73). As well as being told whether your blood group is A, B, AB or O, you will be given a Rhesus blood grouping, either positive or negative. Special attention is given to Rhesus negative mothers. Rhesus negativity is much less common than Rhesus positivity—only about 20 percent of the population is Rhesus negative. If your partner has Rhesus positive blood the chances are that you'll carry a Rhesus positive baby.

As a Rhesus negative person, your immune system will perceive Rhesus positive blood as foreign, and if you're exposed to it, for instance by a transfusion, you will develop antibodies to Rhesus

positive blood cells that will kill them. If you have a Rhesus positive baby and blood cells from the baby pass into your circulation, your body will try to destroy them with Rhesus positive antibodies. With your first baby there is little danger because you are being exposed to Rhesus positive blood cells probably for the first time and the level of Rhesus antibodies will be low or even absent. Blood cells may, however, pass between you and the baby during delivery, vaginal bleeding, abdominal injury (such as a road traffic accident), amniocentesis, CVS and external cephalic version (turning a baby who is in the breech position—see p. 204). Danger during subsequent pregnancies can also be insignificant

THE FIRST PREGNANCY   THE MOTHER'S BLOOD   SUBSEQUENT PREGNANCIES

- Rhesus antibodies
- Rhesus negative
+ Rhesus positive

HOW RH INCOMPATIBILITY OCCURS

In the first pregnancy there is rarely a problem as the maternal and fetal bloodstreams do not mix (above left). If some of the baby's Rhesus positive blood cells escape into the maternal blood (above), they react to form Rhesus antibodies (above right). In subsequent pregnancies, Rhesus antibodies may cross the placenta and damage the baby's blood (above) if it is Rhesus positive.

because antibodies may never be formed in large enough quantities. However, at various points during your prenatal care doctors will take the precaution of finding out what level of antibodies is present in your blood. It's known that a certain level of antibodies may damage the developing baby. This level, however, is reached in less than 10 percent of women who are Rhesus negative. Don't be despondent, therefore, if the doctor tells you that you have Rhesus negative blood. In practical terms all it may mean is that you get extra-special medical care.

BEATING RHESUS INCOMPATIBILITY

Rhesus incompatibility in pregnancy is becoming less and less common as the condition is better understood. After any of the risk episodes listed left, you will be given anti-Rhesus globulin (Anti-D). It may also be given twice routinely to pregnant women who are Rhesus negative but have no antibodies, making your baby safe from Rhesus incompatibility whatever the circumstances.

Babies whose mothers have not had this treatment will not come to any harm. You may have an amniocentesis (see p. 80) and if the baby is affected, an intrauterine transfusion may be carried out.

It may be decided that your baby should be born before term, in which case a cesarean section will be done. In a few cases the delivered baby may need a blood tranfusion to replace its own blood cells which have become damaged during pregnancy. Very occasionally all the baby's blood must be exchanged, especially if jaundice is present. Paradoxically your baby will be given Rhesus negative blood though it has Rhesus positive blood itself. Some of your Rhesus antibodies may still be in your baby's body and would further damage Rhesus positive blood if it were transfused. As a Rhesus positive baby cannot produce antibodies to Rhesus negative cells, the transfused blood cells will die over a period of time and be replaced by the baby's own healthy Rhesus positive blood cells.

The transfusion is done very gradually, but in as little as 72 hours your baby will have got rid of all the antibodies that have been passed on from you, and after the third day there is generally no need for any further transfusions to be carried out. Once the Rhesus antibodies and any bilirubin (the yellow pigment that causes jaundice) have been "washed out" of the baby's system, your baby will come to no further harm and grow up to be a perfectly normal, healthy child.

14
Preparing for the birth

By the 36th week of your pregnancy, you should have given up work and be slowing down your social and domestic routines. You may feel frustrated and bored or you may welcome the rest from your work and the travel to and fro or feel energized and want to spring-clean the house from top to bottom. This is the time to check that everything is ready for the new arrival—the room, the clothing, the equipment—and to prepare yourself, your partner and your other children for the birth.

Organizing your home

THERE ARE MANY THINGS you can do to prepare yourself and the household to cover your day-to-day routine and to make life easier for you after the baby is born.

- If you haven't already got one, invest in a tumble drier. It will make the extra work so much easier, especially if you choose cloth diapers.
- Start to neglect certain parts of your domestic life. Allow the nonessentials to slide and don't worry about them.
- Stop doing any housework that involves hard physical effort.
- Make sure that your family realizes that you can't dash around as you used to. Get others to help with errands.
- Try not to worry about things that don't matter. The highest priority is the baby that is growing inside you. Try to judge your pace and don't overdo anything.
- Sound out a reliable neighbor who will help in emergencies.

- If you have a freezer, stock it with staple foods that freeze well, such as bread, butter, soups, casseroles and vegetables.
- Stock up your food cupboard with tins and dried foods and buy in basic essentials such as soap powder, toilet rolls and disposable diapers.

GETTING THE BABY'S ROOM READY

If you have enough space, you can give the baby a separate room and make it into a nursery, but this isn't absolutely necessary—your baby's space can be a corner of a larger room. Even if you have planned a nursery, you'll probably find you hardly use it in the early weeks after

FURNISHING THE NURSERY
It's a good idea to start with essential items like a crib and bedding, then add other furniture when you have the practical experience of handling your baby.

delivery. You'll find it much more convenient to have your baby with you in your bedroom, particularly at night, and close by you in his bassinett or crib the rest of the time. After these early weeks, it is ideal to have a room that is specially designed and equipped for all your baby's routines, such as feeding, bathing, changing, dressing and playing.

There is no need to go to a lot of expense. Your baby will grow quickly and soon require different things, so there is little point in investing a great deal of money in baby equipment. Before long you'll be adapting the nursery to a toddler's bedroom. Most of the equipment can be purchased second-hand. Look around in local papers and shop windows or at your baby clinic.

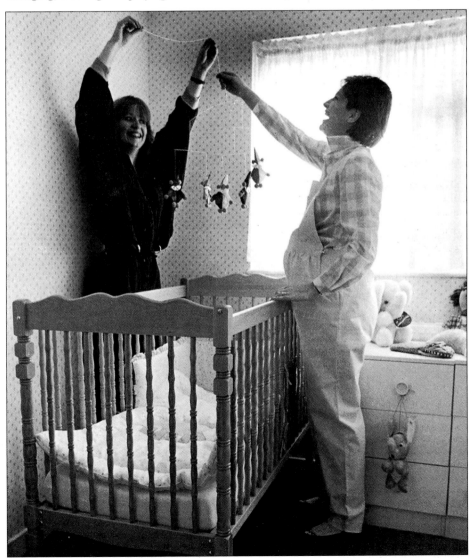

What you need for your baby

IT'S HELPFUL to start thinking about what you need for your baby quite early in your pregnancy, particularly if you're planning any structural changes to your home.

NURSERY EQUIPMENT

• Crib and bassinett—a crib is a luxury for the first few months. Your baby can just as easily sleep in a Moses basket. A tiny baby can sleep in a full-size bassinett provided you do not impede air circulation with a bumper and you lie him down "feet to foot"—so that his feet are touching the foot of the bassinett and he cannot wriggle down under the blankets.

• Moses basket—this can be useful for up to six months depending on the size and vigor of your baby. It can be used as an alternative crib.

• A rear-facing baby car seat with carry handles that can be secured to the back seat of the car.

• For the crib or bassinett, choose a firm, flat mattress with a waterproof cover. Babies should never have pillows as they might suffocate in the fabric covers.

• Cotton fitted sheets or flannelette for warmth—at least 4–5.

• Only use cotton cellular blankets; wool may make him too hot. Duvets should not be used for babies under 12 months.

ESSENTIAL BABY CLOTHING

• 6 stretch suits—you may be showered with tiny clothes for the baby. The first size only lasts about 6 weeks but you will need several because of frequent soiling.

• 2 nightgowns—these make diaper changing easy.

• 4 undershirts—envelope necks are best.

• 2 sweaters or jumpers—avoid lacy patterns which are impractical as they catch around little fingers.

• 2 pairs cotton socks or bootees.

• 1 bonnet or knit cap.

• Cloth squares for catching spit-up and protecting your clothing during burping sessions. They can also be stretched across the crib under the baby's head to catch any spit-up and protect the sheet.

• Diapers—you can opt for reusable diapers or disposables, or a combination of the two. Studies have shown that when diapers, cleansing solution and electricity for the washing machine are added up, disposables are not that much more expensive. You must decide. Use disposables for the first few weeks to give yourself a break from the washing. If you use cotton diapers, buy at least two dozen of good-quality diapers, either shaped diapers with Velcro fastenings or cotton squares with separate diaper pins. You will also need two plastic buckets with lids, and cleansing solution.

• Diaper liners—disposable liners are useful inside cloth diapers as they can contain stools and thus reduce staining.

• At least six pairs of plastic pants if you are using cloth diapers. They quickly become brittle and crack. So buy the best quality and try to wash them by hand.

• Baby bath—this is useful as it means you can bath your baby in the warmest place, not necessarily in the bathroom. It's best to wait till your baby is about four months old before using the big bath.

• Plastic or terry cloth changing pad.

• Two soft new towels for the baby's use—your own towels will feel like sandpaper against the baby's perfect skin.

• Baby bath solution or baby soap.

• Natural sponge or soft facecloths.

• Cotton wool.

• Vaseline, cleansing lotion, toilet rolls or baby wipes for changing time.

• Arachis oil or olive oil for flaky skin.

• Blunt-ended scissors.

• A changing bag—it unfolds to reveal a waterproof area for changing the baby and has pockets all around that hold diapers, change of clothes, cleansing lotion and diaper pins. It can then be rolled up and

slung over your shoulder after the change.
• Baby carriage or stroller—you will have to do a lot of research here to decide on your needs. If you have a car and drive everywhere, a carriage with collapsible frame is perfect. If you travel on public transport, a stroller that collapses easily and adjusts to the horizontal position is ideal. There are so many designs now, so shop around and ask other parents.
• Sling and backpack—the sling is for the first six months or so, depending on the weight of the baby, but a backpack for an older baby can also be useful, especially for a baby who has become accustomed to being carried around.
• Feeding equipment if you are not breastfeeding, or if you express milk for someone else to feed to your baby.

NURSERY FLOOR PLAN
Work out your own requirements by drawing up a floor plan of your baby's room to scale. Make sure that you take account of the position of doors, windows, radiators, and electric sockets and switches.

• A bouncing chair—in this reclining seat the baby can be partly propped up and can see you moving around the room.

ARRANGING A NURSERY

See that all the surfaces in the nursery are hygienic and easy to wipe clean. Make sure that there is plenty of storage space, especially around the changing area. Open shelves for storage mean that it is easy to reach your baby's belongings, but floor-level cupboards will need baby locks later on when your baby becomes more mobile and inquisitive.

Fit a washable floor covering and a dimmer switch for night feeds. Heat control is also important; the temperature should be constant at around 65–68°F (18–20°C), so your baby is neither too hot nor too cold. For your comfort you'll need a low feeding chair and a table. It may be a bit of a luxury, but if it's possible, install a small sink with running water in the corner of the room.

Crib | Low nursing chair | Table for feeding equipment | Nonslip rug | Cupboard | Bath on stand | Sink near changing area and bath | Changing pad | Storage shelves | Diapers

Getting ready for the birth

THE HOSPITAL OR YOUR MIDWIFE will give you a list of the items you will need for the birth. If you are having your baby at home, you will need to prepare a room for the birth.

PREPARING FOR A HOME BIRTH

There are some useful ways you can make your home birth comfortable for yourself and convenient for the midwife.

● Make sure your bed is firm so that you have something to push against and you can avoid getting a puddle of amniotic fluid under your hips. If necessary, put a board under the mattress. You may decide

not to use the bed but have it ready so that all your options are open.

● The most convenient way to make the bed is as follows. Make it up with fresh sheets. Put on a plastic sheet (an old shower curtain will do) and cover with clean old linens. In this way the old sheets and plastic can be taken off after the birth, leaving you in a freshly made bed.

● Provide polythene sheeting to protect furniture and flooring in the room in which you are going to give birth.

● Prepare a work area, such as a table top or a dressing table, that is within easy reach of the bed for supplies.

● The maternity pack provided by the

EQUIPMENT FOR A HOME BIRTH

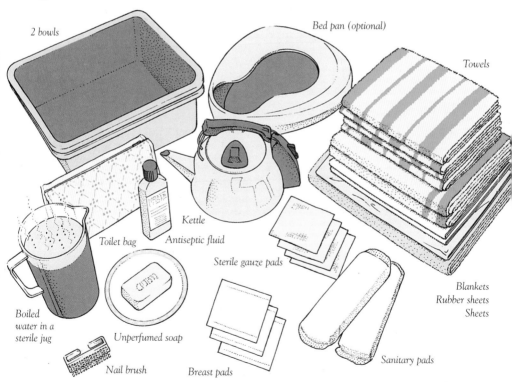

2 bowls

Bed pan (optional)

Towels

Kettle

Toilet bag   Antiseptic fluid

Sterile gauze pads

Boiled water in a sterile jug

Unperfumed soap

Blankets
Rubber sheets
Sheets

Nail brush

Breast pads

Sanitary pads

AIDS FOR LABOR

For hospital delivery your partner or birth assistant will also need to pack a small bag with aids for the labor. Prepare and take with you a bag containing:
- a small natural sponge to moisten her mouth
- Lipbalm or Vaseline to prevent her lips from becoming chapped
- frozen picnic freezing pack or hot water bottle to put against her back if she has bad backache
- a vacuum flask of diluted fruit juice or water (check if the hospital allows) for her to sip during labor
- drinks and sandwiches for yourself and enough left over for her if after delivery she's just missed a meal
- books, playing cards, scrabble, jigsaws, cassette player and tapes to occupy you both while you're waiting between contractions
- coins for the hospital phone box
- leg warmers or thick socks if she starts to shiver during the later stages (see p. 181)
- facecloth to mop her face if she becomes too hot.

midwife before the birth will contain many of the items necessary for the birth. Check with your midwife to see if she will bring a sterile sheet.
- Clear a large area if you plan to have a mobile labor. Have some freshly ironed sheets nearby in case you prefer to deliver on the floor when the time comes.
- To prepare yourself you should have a bath, or a shower to avoid infection if the waters have broken. Otherwise, wash your hands to beyond the wrists, wash your thighs 12 in. (30 cm) down either side, wash the pubic area, all with antiseptic soap, and dry with a clean towel, sterile cloth or gauze pad.
- Have ready a clean nightdress, sanitary pads and underpants for yourself, and a cotton cellular blanket, a disposable diaper and a nightdress or stretch suit for the baby. Prepare the crib with the baby's bedding and blankets in place.

WHAT TO TAKE TO THE HOSPITAL

Several weeks before your baby is due, pack your hospital case with all the things you will need for your stay there. Ask the hospital if they provide a clothes list. Few hospitals provide baby clothes during your stay, though most provide diapers and bedding. You may find that your partner has to fetch and carry clean and soiled clothing during your stay, and then will have to bring in day clothes for you and something

for the baby to wear when you are discharged from the hospital. Remember to set aside loose-fitting clothes. Your breasts will have increased greatly in size when the milk comes in (see p. 221) and your abdomen won't have gone down yet.

FOR YOU

- 2–3 front-opening nightgowns
- 2–3 maternity bras (see p. 137)
- breast pads
- bathrobe
- slippers
- 4 pairs of pants
- sanitary pads – get the most absorbent you can find for the first few days until the lochia subsides (see p. 219)
- toilet bag and contents – hair brush, 2 towels, 2 facecloths
- makeup, face and hand cream and shampoo
- mirror
- coins or card for the telephone

FOR THE BABY

You are likely to need:
- car seat
- 3 undershirts
- 3 stretch suits or onesies
- cotton cellular blanket

Involving your other children

IF YOU HAVE A FAMILY, every member should be involved in your pregnancy. Children should be informed about what is going on and how the pregnancy is progressing, according to their age and how much information they can absorb and understand. Even a very young child will notice that your abdomen is swelling and will want to know why. Give an honest and accurate answer and let your child feel the baby kicking inside you. If your child or children are old enough, put a chart up on the wall of what happens to you and the baby in pregnancy and follow it through as your pregnancy progresses.

If you are having a home confinement you must decide whether you want your children to be involved or not. It is sensible not to restrict the child and if he follows your pregnancy through, the experience will be an enlightening one. Don't be surprised, though, if he gets bored at the time and wants to go off and play. Someone responsible must be there, besides your partner, to take care of him during the labor.

Run through everything with him, especially the fact that it is a bit painful and you are likely to call out, otherwise he may be frightened. You should also prepare him for the birth of the placenta, which is often the bloodiest part. Warn him that you won't be able to answer his questions because you'll be busy and that if the midwife asks him to leave the room, he must do as she says and not hesitate.

If you are going into a hospital, explain to your child what is going to happen and what arrangements will be made, as long

KEEPING YOUR CHILDREN INFORMED
Chart the progress of your pregnancy with your older children and involve them with it as much as possible so they understand what is happening.

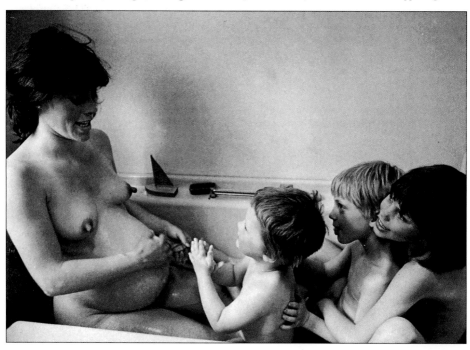

as he is old enough to understand. Even if you will be in a hospital for a short time, say 24 or 48 hours, you will have to make arrangements for someone to take care of your child. If you possibly can, ask someone he knows well to come and look after him in his own home so that his normal routine isn't disrupted too much and he has all his familiar objects around him. If this isn't possible and he has to be looked after in someone else's home, make sure it's somewhere with which he is familiar and where he has spent the night more than once well before the birth— you may have a long labor and so it could be 18–24 hours before your partner is able to collect him.

Make sure that your child knows exactly how long you are likely to be apart. Prepare him in other ways by pointing out small babies to him; show him pictures of his own babyhood and relate this to the coming arrival. Buy him a doll of his own so that he feels he has a baby too. It helps too if your partner increases his involvement with the child, particularly with the usual routines of bathing, feeding and storytelling.

If your child is old enough to understand, it will help if you can rehearse what is going to happen so that he becomes familiar with the future events. It is surprise that will upset him. Compile a timetable of what you will do when labor starts and go over this with him in detail so he becomes familiar with the scenario. If you rehearse the whole scheme together several times he will feel happy and secure in the knowledge that you are taking special care of him.

COUNTDOWN FOR LABOR

Home confinement
1 Call the midwife.
2 Call your partner or birth assistant.
3 Contact whoever is caring for your other children and alert them.
4 Make yourself a hot drink.
5 Check that the room is ready.
6 Have a hot bath or shower.

Hospital confinement
1 Call the hospital, then call an ambulance or taxi if you are not being driven in by your partner or a friend. Don't drive yourself.
2 Call your partner or birth assistant.
3 Alert whoever is caring for your children that you are going in.
4 Make yourself a hot drink.
5 Collect together your handbag, coat and your packed bag.
6 Sit down and wait for your partner or the ambulance.

If someone is driving you to the hospital, you should know how to get there and how long it will take. Plot an alternative route in case the traffic is heavy or you find the road blocked for some reason. Whenever possible, choose well-made roads so that your journey will be comfortable. Find out which hospital entrance you should use, during the day and night, to get you to the ward by the most direct route. Make sure you and the driver are thoroughly familiar with all this information and, if it puts your mind at rest, do a trial run.

Signs of labor
In the week or two before you go into labor you may experience signs that something is about to happen.
1 You feel a "lightening" or engagement, when the baby's head drops into the pelvis.
2 The baby's engagement causes an increase in pressure on the bladder and you will find that you want to pass urine more frequently again.
3 Braxton Hicks contractions become more frequent and may get stronger.
4 Often vaginal secretions increase a day or so before labor starts. If it's your first baby you may have a "show" (see p. 30) as much as two weeks before labor.
5 You may notice slight weight loss in the last week.
6 Some women experience a nesting instinct, wanting to clean the house.

15

Labor and birth

This is the high point to which all your preparations during pregnancy have been leading. While it would be unrealistic to expect the birth to be pain-free, you can hope for it to be relaxed and happy.

You will be pleased, despite the discomfort, if everything and everyone around you are known to you. You will be relaxed if you understand what is happening to you and are confident that you can control your body and help during the delivery. If you learn about labor and birth and practice the exercises and breathing techniques, you should feel less pain and be alert to enjoy giving birth.

Labor

LABOR CAN BE DIVIDED into well-defined stages. There is a stage before labor begins, sometimes called pre-labor. The first labor stage is divided into two; the early phase is when you start going into labor and when contractions may be short, irregular and not too painful. This culminates in the late first stage of labor and the transition when your contractions become regular, more frequent and painful and result in full dilatation of the cervix. The second stage of labor is when you push the baby through the birth canal and it ends with the birth of your baby. Labor is not complete until you have gone through the third stage, which is delivery of the placenta (afterbirth).

PAIN IN LABOR

Every woman feels the pain of contractions differently but in early labor they may be similar to menstrual cramps and sometimes they're confined to mild backache. The kind of labor that proceeds well into the first stage with nothing more than gradually worsening backache is often called back labor (see p. 181). Very often a contraction feels like a wave of discomfort across your abdomen that reaches a crescendo for a few seconds and then diminishes. At the same time you can feel a hardening and tightening of the uterine muscle, which is held at the peak of its intensity for a few seconds and then begins to relax. You have no control over your contractions—they are "involuntary"—though your state of mind during labor can have a profound effect on contractions, making them feel more or less painful.

Most women assume that contractions will get longer, more frequent and stronger in a steady pattern. This is not so and don't be disturbed if your contractions seem to vary. It is absolutely normal for a strong contraction, for example, to be followed by a weaker one that doesn't last quite as long. It is also normal for contractions to follow one another relentlessly—this is more likely if labor has been induced and is kept going with an intravenous drip (see pp. 200–201).

Onset of Labor

Most people think the onset of labor will be very clear; pains will come, contractions will start and you'll know. It often isn't clear at all. Three things might happen, though they don't necessarily mean that birth is imminent.
● The blood-tinged, gelatinous plug of mucus that has blocked the cervical canal may be dislodged during the early first stage of labor (although this can happen as much as two weeks beforehand), and always precedes rupture of the membranes. It is sometimes called the show and means that the cervix is beginning to stretch.
● Your membranes may rupture at any time up to the delivery. Leakage of the amniotic fluid varies from being a gush to a slight dribble that can be stemmed by wearing a sanitary pad. There is no pain accompanying rupture of the membranes and the flow depends on the site and size of the break and whether or not the baby's

LENGTH OF LABOR

Labor is usually longest with a first baby, an average 12–14 hours. Thereafter labor lasts an average seven hours. In general, the lighter the contractions, the longer the labor will be. A fast labor tends to start with long, slow contractions and proceeds in the same way.

head can plug the hole. If the membranes have ruptured you should contact the midwife or the hospital immediately.
● You may feel a dull backache or, if you had Braxton Hicks contractions during the third trimester, you may mistake the early contractions of labor for stronger Braxton Hicks. Severe Braxton Hicks can be mistaken for labor, however, and this is known as a "false labor." Time these early contractions over an hour and if they get closer together and longer in duration, you're probably in labor. The intervals between contractions once it's established that you're in labor are timed from the end of one to the beginning of the next. The contractions tend to be 30–60 seconds long at first, building up gradually to 75 seconds during the most active phase of labor.

THE PRESENTATION

The presenting part of your baby is the part that will be born first. Most babies lie in a well-flexed (curled-up) position with the chin resting on the chest (near right). The way the baby presents can affect labor and birth; a posterior presentation (far right) can lead to an erratic backache labor (see p. 181). If the face is presenting, labor may be slower and the baby's features may be slightly swollen for about 24 hours.

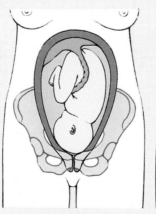 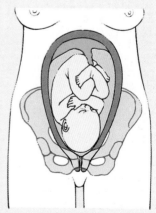

WELL-FLEXED POSITION   POSTERIOR PRESENTATION

ADMISSION TO A HOSPITAL

When you reach the labor ward the midwife will prepare you for the birth. Your birth attendant can stay with you while she does this.

● She will consult your notes and ask you about how the labor has progressed so far—whether your waters have gone, how frequently the contractions are coming and whether or not you have moved your bowels.

● You will be asked to undress and to change into the loose-fitting nightdress,

INITIAL EXAMINATION
When you arrive in the maternity unit, a doctor or midwife will gently feel your abdomen so that she can establish which way the baby is facing.

T-shirt or gown that you have brought with you to wear for the labor and birth.

● You will be examined; the midwife will palpate your abdomen to feel the baby's position, she will listen to the fetal heartbeat, take your blood pressure, pulse and temperature, and you'll be given an internal examination to see how far your cervix has dilated.

● You will be asked to give a urine sample to test for protein and sugar.

● You can then have a shower or bath if you like, and make yourself comfortable in the delivery room with the help of your birth partner and the midwife. If you have any questions or you want to discuss your birthplan (see p. 240) and make your feelings known to the staff, now is the time to remind them of your preferences.

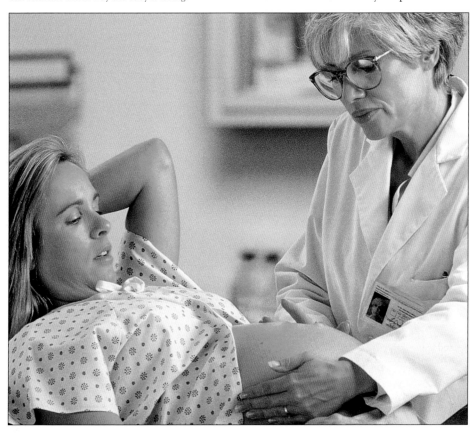

BREATHING FOR LABOR AND BIRTH

If you have practiced a relaxation technique (see p. 143) and have learned to recognize the different types or levels of breathing, now is the time to put them into practice. Your birth assistant will be able to help you by reminding you when your breathing is too rapid or your shoulders are tense. The birth assistant can help by tapping out a rhythm or using words like "breath, breath, pant, pant, blow."

EARLY FIRST STAGE
The contractions in the early stages will probably be gentle and you should be able to breathe deeply and evenly throughout. Greet each contraction with a slow, even breath out.

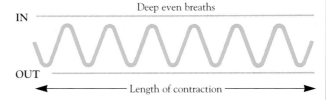

LATE FIRST STAGE
Take your opening breath out and then try to breathe above the contractions; light, short breaths that hardly seem to involve the lower parts of your body at all. Take a deep breath and relax when it is all over, to signal to yourself and those around you that the contraction is over.

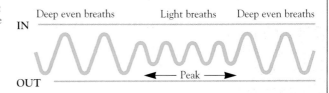

TRANSITIONAL STAGE
If you want to push too early, try the shallowest breathing of all—panting—though without hyperventilating and starving your body of carbon dioxide. Breathe only in your mouth. If you feel dizzy, your birth assistant can cup his hands over your nose and mouth while you are breathing.

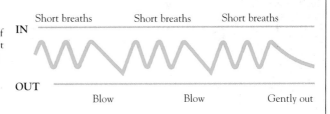

SECOND STAGE
This should be the most natural pattern of breathing for you. Take a deep breath and hold it while bearing down and letting your pelvic floor bulge outward. Let your push be long and smooth. Then repeat if the contraction is still intense; relax when it ends.

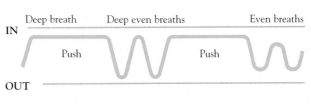

The first stage of labor

DURING THIS STAGE the cervix opens out (dilates) to allow the baby's head to pass through. Before it dilates, the cervix becomes thinned and softened and is gradually pulled up by the contracting uterine muscle. This is called effacement. The muscle of the upper segment of the uterus contracts and puts pressure on the lower segment, which in turn transmits the pull of the contractions to the cervix. As a result, once the cervix has stretched, it dilates with each contraction until the entire cervical canal is eliminated. You are then fully dilated. The degrees of dilatation of the cervix have been standardized so that it can be described

accurately and progress can be charted. If you ask the midwife how labor is progressing, she will probably respond in terms of the number of centimeters of cervical dilatation or perhaps with the number of fingers (one finger is about one centimeter). Dilatation is normally given in one-centimeter increments up to four centimeters. At five or six centimeters the cervix is described as dilated. When the cervix is said to be fully dilated it is approximately 10 centimeters in diameter. This is the completion of the first stage of labor, though in real terms the first stage often moves gradually and smoothly into the second stage without punctuation.

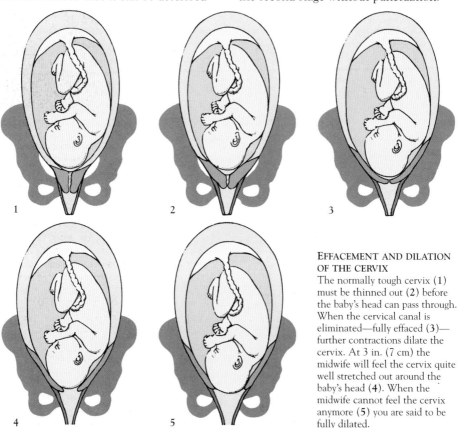

EFFACEMENT AND DILATION OF THE CERVIX
The normally tough cervix (1) must be thinned out (2) before the baby's head can pass through. When the cervical canal is eliminated—fully effaced (3)— further contractions dilate the cervix. At 3 in. (7 cm) the midwife will feel the cervix quite well stretched out around the baby's head (4). When the midwife cannot feel the cervix anymore (5) you are said to be fully dilated.

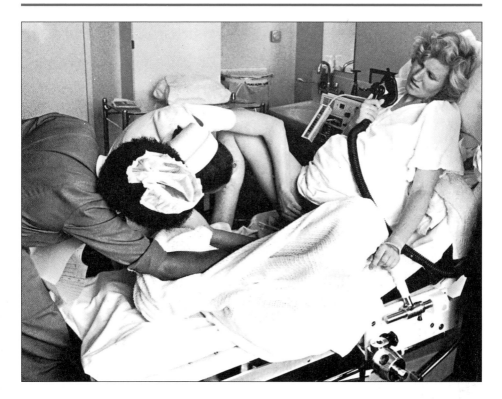

EXAMINATIONS DURING LABOR

If you have asked for an epidural, an anesthetist will visit you after the admission procedure. If not, you will be left with your partner or birth assistant and a nurse or midwife will be with you throughout your labor.

The fetal heart will be regularly monitored either by fetoscope, Doppler or a machine (see p. 202). Internal examinations may be done every four hours to check progress. The midwife will do this while you are sitting up or lying on your side on the bed, or even standing if it's more comfortable for you. Let her know which position you prefer.

The midwife who examines you will almost certainly be one of the team who has been looking after you throughout. She will let you know that it is time to examine you and will tell you how things are progressing. Ask her, or get your

ASSESSING PROGRESS
Your caregivers will check how far your cervix has dilated and will tell you how well you are doing.

partner to ask her, if you don't understand something. If you feel that your contractions are getting longer and stronger and you haven't had an internal examination for a while, then ask for one. It is quite cheering to find that your cervical dilatation has progressed between examinations.

It is possible that your companion will be asked to leave during your preparation and any internal examinations. This is absolutely unnecessary—people who have nothing to do with your birth will be coming into the room all the time—so make sure that your companion stays.

You may be asked questions during an internal examination or while you are having a contraction. Concentrate on what you are doing and answer the question when the contraction is over.

ADVICE TO BIRTH ASSISTANT

● During prelabor, encourage her to sleep and to conserve her strength. You may see a burst of energy, which is the nesting instinct, but do tell her firmly to rest and put her feet up as much as possible.

● In the early stages of labor and if the membranes haven't ruptured, encourage her to take a warm bath and help her to get in and out of the bath so that she doesn't slip. If the membranes have ruptured, a shower is best (see p. 169).

● Unless she is feeling nauseous, encourage her to eat and drink as she wants. Natural fruit juice and honey contain sugars which will give her plenty of energy. You should try to have something to eat too, as there may not be time later.

● When the contractions begin you should time them and note the interval between them (from the end of one to the beginning of another) and how long each contraction lasts. Put your hand on her abdomen so that you can feel the peak of the contraction.

● One of your most important roles is to coach her through the contractions, giving comfort and support. Never criticize; use positive words and praise as much as you can. Don't be offended if she turns away from you and seeks reassurance from the midwife. She is seeking help from the experienced woman and not rejecting you.

● She will find it very soothing if you wipe her face. Your touch is comforting—try massaging her back or her abdomen gently, or just hold hands.

● Be on the watch for any signs of tension in her neck, shoulders and forehead and remind her to relax and tell her how to do it. It's a good idea for her to keep her mouth loose between contractions, so if you see any signs of tension encourage her to close her mouth and drop her jaw.

● If she is up and mobile, remind her to empty her bladder every hour. If she gets up and moves about, stay near her because any kind of activity can increase the contractions. Go with her when she goes to the toilet, and stay with her in the cubicle.

● Observe her moods and fit in with them. If she wants to stay quiet, then do so, but if she wants to be distracted, play a game of cards or Scrabble.

● When you arrive at the hospital and she is having contractions, simply sign the essential forms and go directly to the labor ward. Any other forms can be filled out later. The most important thing is to move her as little as possible and get her settled as comfortably and as quickly as you can. Try to prevent anything in the hospital making her anxious or distracting from her control of her labor.

● You'll be able to stay with your partner during the admissions procedure, but if things are still in the very early stages, this might be a good time to slip out for a bite to eat. Your partner is going to need you with her all the time later on.

● If the medical staff suggest painkilling drugs, make sure that she knows what is being offered and what they are for. If she feels like trying to hang on, help her do so, but you should always remember that there is absolutely no reason why she should not be given drugs if they are medically indicated in her case. If she asks for pain relief, don't discourage her unduly— remember that she is the one in labor, and it is her decision.

● If you're at home, the midwife will probably be on her own for most of the time, so be ready to assist whenever she asks. Do as she says quickly.

● When labor is well established, you could place your hand on her abdomen so that you can feel it begin to tighten and know when the next contraction is coming. As the uterus starts to harden and rise, tell her to take in a deep breath. You can make sure that she is not caught off-guard by contractions and therefore she will be able to control them better.

LOVING SUPPORT
Touching and stroking at any time during labor are immensely helpful.

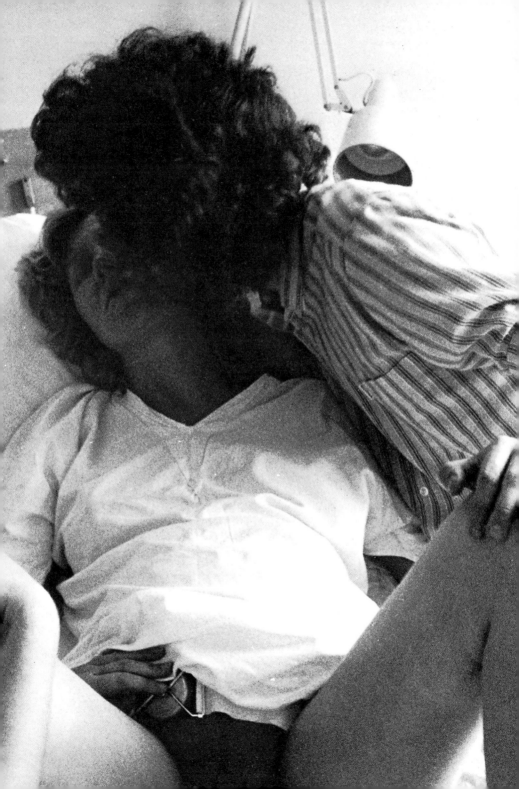

POSITIONS FOR THE FIRST STAGE

There is no single "correct" position for labor; you need to experiment and find the most comfortable position for you. Move around and keep trying new positions. You can use the furniture or your partner for support if you like. Many women like to move around and when the contraction starts, take up their chosen position.

STAYING UPRIGHT
This encourages contractions during the first stage. You will feel more comfortable if your knees are slightly apart and your back is straight. Use a cushion over the back of a chair to lean against.

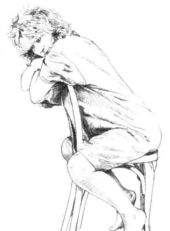

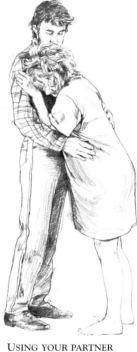

IN THE VERY EARLY STAGES OF LABOR
Stop what you are doing during the contraction and support yourself on whatever is close by. If the surface is high, kneel down and lean slightly forward.

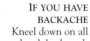

USING YOUR PARTNER
Lean onto your birth assistant. The weight of the baby will be taken off your spine and the contractions will be most efficient in this upright position. He can massage your back.

IF YOU HAVE BACKACHE
Kneel down on all fours and rock backwards and forwards during contractions. Don't arch your back—lean forward between contractions onto your folded arms or sit back on your haunches.

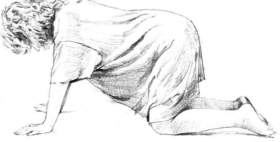

THE TRANSITIONAL STAGE

This is the period from the end of the first stage of labor to the beginning of the second stage. Not all women experience it as a well-defined, distinct stage of labor, but some do and it is as well to be prepared. It rarely lasts for more than an hour, often much less, but it can be quite hard to cope with. Coming at the end of several hours in the first stage, some women become discouraged and feel that they can't go on without pain relief. There may be some shaking and shivering, which is physiological and not abnormal. Simply because of all the hormone changes that are going on you may feel some irritability and ill-temper and some women feel so nauseous that they want to vomit. Don't resist this urge because you will feel a lot better afterwards. You may feel excited and restless; every position seems uncomfortable. You may feel anxious for your own safety and for the baby's, and you may feel sleepy between contractions because most of the oxygen in your body is being taken up by the uterus and the baby, and your brain is relatively short of it.

Some women feel the urge to push during this stage but don't bear down until it is confirmed that you are fully dilated. If you feel a strong urge to push but it is too soon to do so, use the panting and blowing breathing technique (see p. 144) until the midwife tells you it is safe to start to push.

ADVICE TO BIRTH ASSISTANT

- Try to get her to relax. Refrain from asking questions and remove perspiration if she's sweating a lot.
- If she tells you not to touch her, refrain but stay near the bed. If she feels sick and wants to vomit, get a basin and encourage her to do so. Always praise her.
- If her legs start to tremble, put on her socks and hold her legs firmly.
- If you notice that she is beginning to grunt and make pushing movements, let the midwife know immediately. This is a difficult time for your partner, and you can encourage her by explaining that you think she is in transition, stage two is beginning and the baby will soon be born.
- You will know that the delivery is imminent when the midwife says that the head is crowning—it is beginning to emerge from the vaginal opening.

For most women the end of the transition stage is marked by a noticeable change in the pattern of breathing. You may grunt involuntarily, and this is because you will start to feel the urge to bear down. The need to push becomes very strong. Do tell your assistant to alert the staff that you are ready to push. They will confirm that the cervix has dilated 10 centimeters and the second stage is beginning. Your baby is about to be born.

BACK LABOR

If your baby is in the posterior position, its head may be pressing against your sacrum. This usually results in a long, erratic labor accompanied by backache. In this position the baby's head is not properly flexed and a wider part presents. However, the baby usually rotates before passing through the birth canal and the birth itself is normal. If your backache is particularly bad, there are ways to relieve it.

- Keep moving, and during contractions take up a position in which the pressure is taken off your back, for example on all fours, leaning into a chair, or rocking to and fro.
- Nullify the pressure with counterpressure. Your birth assistant can apply pressure with fists or something round such as a tennis ball against your back.
- Apply a hot water bottle to the lower part of your back between contractions.
- Don't lie flat on your back; the baby's head then presses onto your spine.
- Massage the buttocks and the lower back (see p. 145).

POSITIONS DURING THE TRANSITION

Transition is a difficult stage in which to find a comfortable position. Contractions seem relentless but if you understand that the baby will be born soon, that should give you the encouragement and confidence to stay calm and patient. You probably won't feel like moving around so much but try to change positions every now and again.

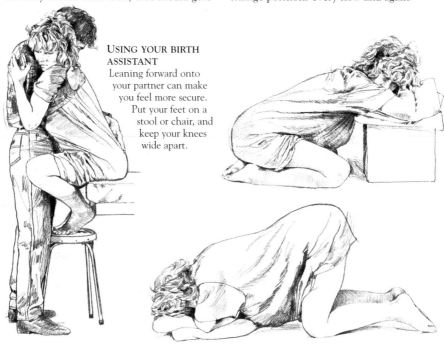

USING YOUR BIRTH ASSISTANT
Leaning forward onto your partner can make you feel more secure. Put your feet on a stool or chair, and keep your knees wide apart.

IF THE CERVIX IS NOT FULLY DILATED
If you feel the need to bear down, use gravity to slow the baby down while the cervix continues to dilate. Kneel down and either sit back on your haunches and rest your head in your arms against a low chair, or lean forward and put your head on your arms on the floor and your bottom in the air. This takes pressure off your lower back.

IF YOU WANT TO REST
Lie down on your side with cushions under your head and upper thigh. Keep your legs as wide apart as possible.

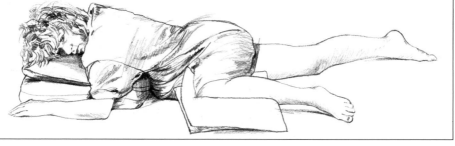

POSITIONS FOR DELIVERY

You will know by now from your experience of labor what position will be most comfortable to give birth in. Take advice from your medical attendants; they will lead you through the pushing stage. Enjoy yourself and take your time.

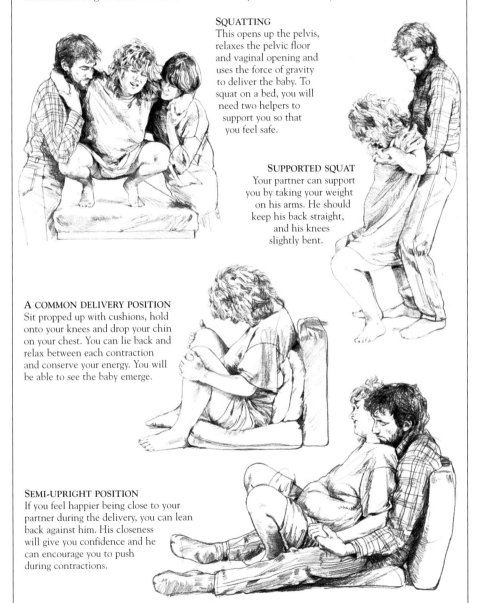

SQUATTING
This opens up the pelvis, relaxes the pelvic floor and vaginal opening and uses the force of gravity to deliver the baby. To squat on a bed, you will need two helpers to support you so that you feel safe.

SUPPORTED SQUAT
Your partner can support you by taking your weight on his arms. He should keep his back straight, and his knees slightly bent.

A COMMON DELIVERY POSITION
Sit propped up with cushions, hold onto your knees and drop your chin on your chest. You can lie back and relax between each contraction and conserve your energy. You will be able to see the baby emerge.

SEMI-UPRIGHT POSITION
If you feel happier being close to your partner during the delivery, you can lean back against him. His closeness will give you confidence and he can encourage you to push during contractions.

The second stage

FOR A FIRST BABY the second stage generally doesn't last longer than two hours—the average is around one hour and it may be as little as 15–20 minutes for subsequent babies. Bearing down is a reflex, an instinctive urge to push down, which is caused by the baby's head pressing on the pelvic floor and the rectum. Even if you know nothing about

ADVICE TO BIRTH ASSISTANT

● Remind her to relax her pelvic floor during pushing. She should take two or three deep breaths and push her hardest at the peak of contractions. She should push in a strong, steady way.

● Remind her to look in the mirror so that she can see the baby emerging.

● If you are in a hospital and are asked to leave the delivery room suddenly, do so without question. There may be a medical emergency and staff will have to move very fast. You cannot guarantee that you will not be in the way. Leave the delivery room but stay close by outside.

● Remind her to lie back and relax fully between contractions so that she conserves her strength for pushing.

● You are now more of an observer once the baby's head has crowned. The midwife will be the one who coaches your partner through the pushing stage.

● Don't expect your partner to communicate with you during the birth. She will be preoccupied and may not notice you for some time.

● When the baby is placed on your partner's stomach, if possible put your arms around them both to keep them warm and signal that you're still there.

● Be ready for your own and your partner's reactions. There may be tears, silence, whoops of joy, perhaps even squeamishness. It's all perfectly normal and understandable so don't feel you have to hold back your emotions.

the mechanics of labor you will know automatically to take a deep breath, so lowering your diaphragm which exerts pressure on the uterus and helps the pushing. You then hold your breath, slightly bend your knees and strain downwards. Pushing is instinctive. It doesn't hurt the baby but it is quite hard work, and much harder work if you are lying on your back because you actually have to push the baby uphill (see p. 64). It is much less difficult if you are in an upright position, squatting, sitting up supported, on all fours, or on your knees leaning against a chair or your partner. This way you have the force of gravity to help you. Your pushing should be smooth and continuous. All of the muscular effort should be down and out. It should be fairly slow and gradual so that the vaginal tissues and muscles are given time to stretch and accommodate your baby's head without tearing or making an episiotomy necessary.

You should push during a contraction. Your pushing effort only *helps* the uterus to expel the baby. The involuntary muscles of the uterus can expel the baby on their own. So you help most by beginning your pushing effort with the peak intensity of each contraction.

During pushing, the pelvic floor and the anal area should be as relaxed as possible, so make a conscious effort to relax this part of your body (see p. 125). You may lose a little stool but don't be embarrassed. Don't worry about urinating either; it is very common. When you've finished a push you will find two slow, deep breaths helpful, but don't relax too quickly at the end of each contraction as the baby will maintain its forward progress if you relax slowly.

THE URGE TO PUSH
Pushing is instinctive. Even if you don't understand why, you will automatically take a deep breath and push downwards.

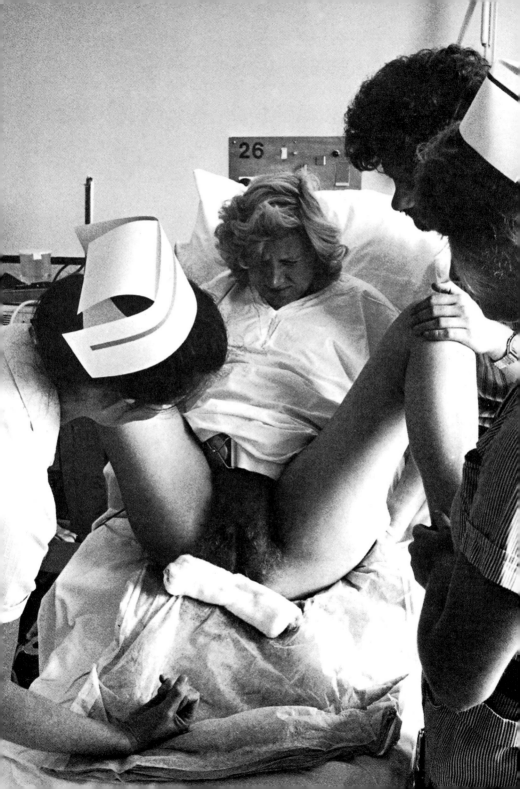

BIRTH

The first sign that the baby is coming is bulging of the anus and perineum. With each contraction more and more of the baby's head appears at the vaginal opening, though it may slip back slightly between contractions. If you're watching in a mirror don't be disheartened—this is normal. After crowning, the head will be delivered in the next contraction or two. You can reach down at this point and touch the head to reassure yourself.

It is normal to feel a stinging or burning sensation as the baby stretches the outlet of the birth canal. As soon as you feel it, stop bearing down, pant and allow the uterus to push the baby out on its own. As you stop pushing, try to go limp. Make a conscious effort to relax the muscles of the perineal floor (see p. 125). The burning or stinging sensation lasts for a short time and is immediately followed by a numb feeling as the baby's head stretches the vaginal tissues so thin that the nerves are blocked, having a natural anesthetic effect. If the medical staff feel you are going to tear badly, this is the moment they may do an episiotomy (see p. 198). As the baby's head is delivered, you will feel a sensation like toothpaste coming out of a tube. Once the head has emerged, the midwife will check that the cord is not around the baby's neck (see p. 191).

When the head is delivered, the baby's back is uppermost; its face is pointing towards your rectum. Almost immediately, however, it will start to rotate its shoulders so that it is facing your right or left thigh. The direction depends on its position in the uterus. The midwife will wipe its eyes, nose and mouth with clean gauze, and remove any fluid from the nose and upper air passages. Now there may be a breathing space when the uterine contractions stop for a few minutes. When they restart, it's hardly necessary for you to push because within the next one or two contractions, the baby's shoulders will be born, followed by its body. Sometimes the head and body are born in the one contraction.

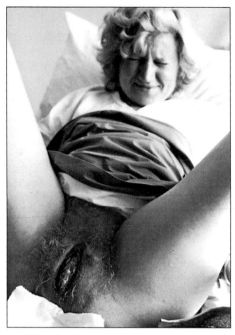

1 With each contraction in the second stage of labor, more of the baby's head appears at the vaginal opening. The anus and the perineum bulge out with the pressure of the head.

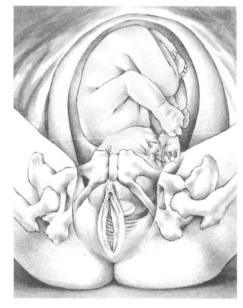

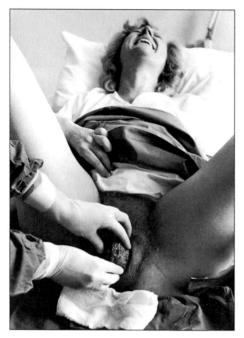

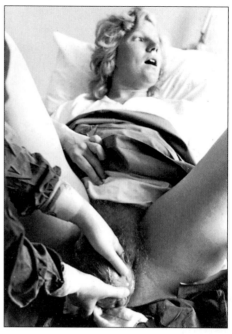

2 As the baby's head crowns, the stinging sensation is followed by numbness as the vaginal tissues are stretched so thin that the nerves are blocked. The head then slips out at last.

3 The baby's head is born facing downwards towards the rectum but the baby immediately turns to face your thigh to get into a good position for the birth of the body.

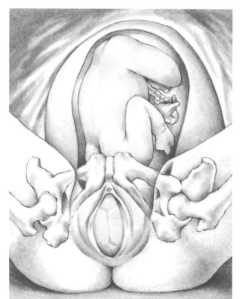

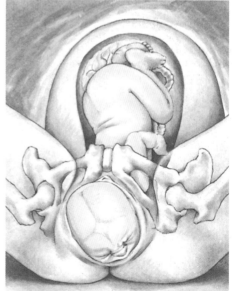

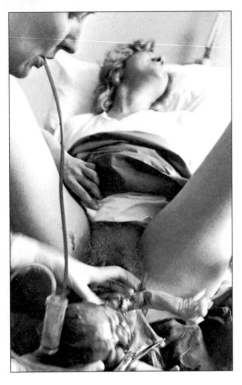

4 The midwife will clear any fluid and mucus from the baby's air passages. The next uterine contraction is usually sufficient to deliver the shoulders and then the body.

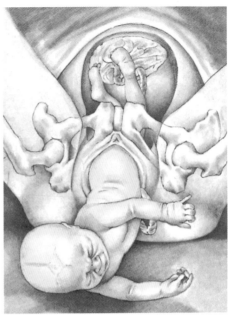

The midwife usually assists this last part of delivery by putting her thumbs and fingers under the armpits of your baby and lifting him upwards towards your abdomen, holding him firmly as he will be slippery with blood and amniotic fluid. If you're feeling alert and you're in a position to do so, you can bend down and pull your baby out yourself and onto your abdomen.

Your baby may cry when first delivered and will be crying lustily a few seconds after birth. If the breathing is normal, there's absolutely no reason why you should not take hold of the baby immediately. Ask if you can lay the baby on your abdomen and keep him warm with your arms and those of your partner. If there's a danger of the baby being cold, all three of you can be kept warm with a warm towel or blanket. Your gentle stroking movements, your soothing voice and the sound of your heartbeat are all right for your baby.

Your baby will probably be a bluish color at first and may be covered with the white greasy vernix (see p. 87). He will have streaks of blood on his head and body and depending on your delivery his head may be elongated after the journey down the birth canal. The midwife will make a check of his general condition (see p. 218). If there is fluid in the mouth or nose or air passages, the midwife will want to make sure that it's cleared and breathing is normal. She will suck it out. If the baby doesn't start to breathe immediately, the midwife will take him and give him oxygen. Don't be alarmed at the sudden activity. As soon as the baby's breathing is normal, he will be returned to you to hold.

5 The baby is born and handed to the mother while the cord is clamped and eventually cut. The uterus will soon begin to contract again to expel the placenta, accelerated if necessary with an injection.

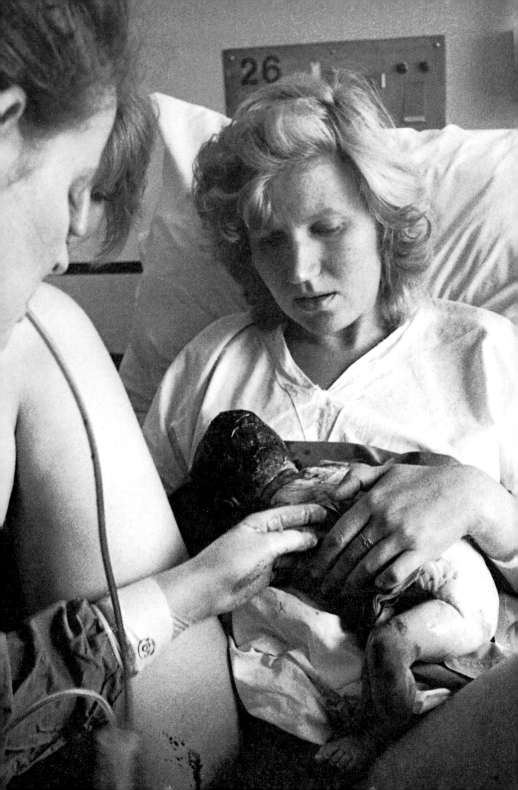

The third stage

WHEN THE BABY IS BORN the uterus rests and after about 15 minutes starts to contract comparatively painlessly again to expel the placenta. This is the third stage of labor. When the head appears the midwife usually gives the mother an injection in the thigh of syntometrine or ergometrine, a synthetic hormone that increases the contractions of the uterus and expels the placenta more quickly than would happen normally. Oxytocin, produced naturally in response to seeing and touching your baby, but most of all to putting him to the breast, does the same job as ergometrine, but ergometrine is usually administered in hospital, although the midwife or doctor will ask you first.

In the third stage of labor the placenta detaches itself from the uterine wall. The large blood vessels, about the thickness of a pencil, that run to and from the placenta are simply torn across. Most women do not bleed, however, because the muscle fibers of the uterus are arranged in a criss-cross fashion, and when the uterus contracts down, the muscles tighten around the blood vessels, preventing them from bleeding. This is why it's absolutely essential that the uterus contracts down into a hard ball once the placenta has been expelled. The uterus can be kept tightly contracted by massaging it for an hour or so after the third stage is complete.

The placenta slips out with a gentle squelch. It looks rather like a piece of liver and many women like to look at it and examine it. It is an amazing organ—it has been the life support system for your baby for nine months. Once the placenta is delivered, the midwife will examine it to make sure that none of it has been left behind. If any of the placenta has been retained by the uterus it can be a cause of hemorrhage later on (see p. 210).

You may shiver profoundly after delivery of the placenta. After delivery of my second child I was shivering so much and my teeth were chattering so that I couldn't speak and couldn't breathe properly. My explanation for this reaction is that for nine months I had a little furnace inside me, producing a lot of heat, and my body had adjusted to take account of that heat production by turning my own thermostat down slightly. When my baby left my body, I was deprived of that heat and I started shivering to raise my body temperature. The shivering usually passes in about half an hour, during which time the body temperature has been brought back up to normal and your own thermostat reset. Often the muscles in the legs feel quite sore for a day or two.

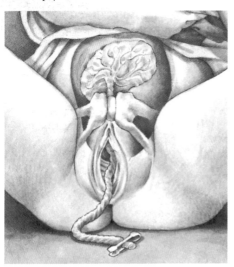

DELIVERY OF THE PLACENTA
When the contractions resume, they will be less painful. One or two pushes should expel the placenta. The midwife will put one hand on your uterus and will gently pull on the cord with the other to ease the placenta out.

CLAMPING THE CORD

There is no need for the unseemly rush to clamp the cord that there used to be 30 years ago when I first qualified. The cord will only need to be clamped and cut

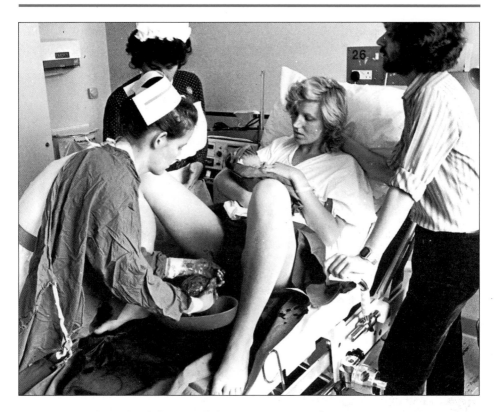

HOLDING YOUR BABY
While the placenta is being expelled, you can hold your baby for the first time.

at once if it is looped tightly around the baby's neck. This is quite common, and the baby will then be delivered very quickly. Usually the midwife will be able to slip the cord out from around the baby's head and the delivery can proceed without immediate clamping. It's generally believed that the baby benefits from the return of placental blood through the umbilical cord and that it should not be clamped until it stops pulsating. (Blood can flow from the placenta to the baby only if the baby is at a lower level than the uterus.) When the time is right, the cord is divided between a pair of clamps placed 5–6 in. (13–15 cm) from the baby's navel.

Now the three of you should be left alone. Put your baby to the breast as soon as possible—preferably in the first five minutes and even before the cord is clamped if that's an option. Breastfeeding releases oxytocin which helps the uterus to contract, and the colostrum in your breasts (see p. 221) contains antibodies that will guard against some forms of gastric infection. Don't worry if he doesn't want to suckle, just concentrate on getting to know him. A newborn is usually alert during the first hour after a normal birth, and will look intently at you if you hold him 8–10 in. (20–25 cm) from your face. He can focus at this distance, which is the distance between your face and his when you cradle him to the breast.

Presently you will be washed, stitched if necessary and asked to pass urine to check that everything is working all right. The midwives will wipe the baby and weigh him and put him in the crib ready for transferral to the postnatal ward.

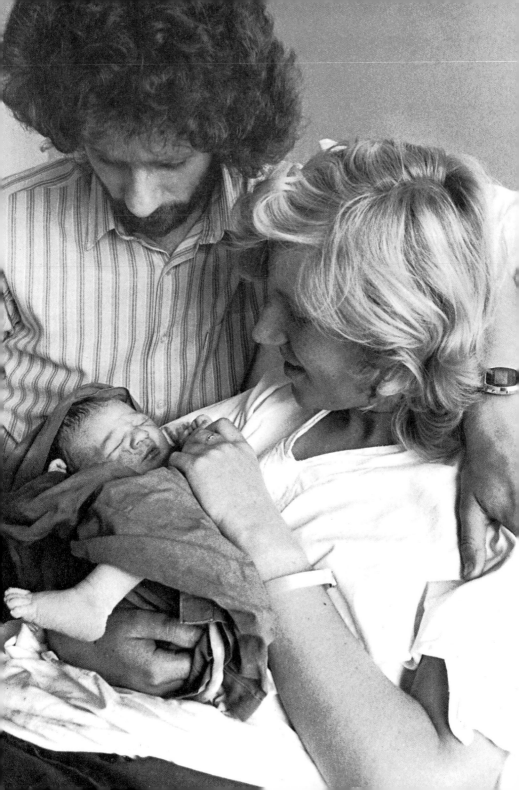

SUDDEN DELIVERY

If you are alone, or if your doctor or midwife has not arrived when the baby is about to be born, try to pant or blow until they arrive. You should be able to keep this up for five minutes even though the urge to push plus the pressure from the baby's head crowning may make it difficult. Whatever you do, don't try to hold your legs together to delay the birth, and don't allow anyone else to do this. If your baby is coming and you cannot comfortably delay it, don't try to interfere. If you are totally alone, sitting on the floor in a semiupright position is probably the safest and most comfortable one for you to be in. Holding onto something firm with your arms is both sensible and efficient. Make sure that your baby is delivered onto something soft and clean (a sheet, large towel or tablecloth would do). If you can manage, you may even help the baby out yourself once the head has been

YOUR BABY IS BORN
You'll never forget this first moment. You'll seem lost in wonder at this little human being, complete with perfect features and tiny hands and feet.

delivered and the shoulders are clear of the vagina. After that sit or lie down with your baby's skin close to your own; your body heat will keep the baby warm. Cover yourselves with a sheet or blanket and put the baby to suckle at your breast while you wait for help to arrive.

SPECIAL CARE BABY UNIT

If there is a problem with the baby, such as low birthweight, he may be taken to the special care baby unit. You may feel disappointed that you can't touch and feed him but the staff will be sympathetic, so ask to be allowed to help with the care of your baby. Don't panic, ask questions and expect answers that help you to understand what is happening. If you find you can't communicate effectively, ask your partner or a friend to talk to the pediatrician, or nurse in charge. You will be encouraged to breastfeed your baby if you want to, even though he is in an incubator. The hospital will supply you with a pump to express your milk for him and it will be fed to him by tube. Touch him as much as you can so that you gain confidence in handling such a tiny baby.

TWINS

Labor is no more painful with a twin delivery than with a single baby. Almost certainly you will be advised to have the babies in hospital in case you need extra help with the birth, if the babies are not presenting properly (see p. 159). There is no reason why your partner shouldn't stay with you during the delivery, and you should discuss the possibility with your midwife during the last trimester. Your consultant will probably recommend an epidural anesthetic (see p. 196) as twin labors can be prolonged.

There is only one first stage of labor if you're having twins. Once the cervix is fully dilated and you're able to push, both babies are pushed out, one after the other. There are two second stages, though the second

one will be short, especially if the second baby is smaller than the first. The majority of second babies are born within 10–30 minutes of the first.

Emotionally a twin birth is different from a single birth. You'll hardly appreciate the delivery of the second baby, such is the feeling of triumph and joy when the first baby is born. Once the first baby is born, the midwife will examine you to see how the second baby is lying. The contractions will begin again after a few minutes and the membranes will be artificially ruptured. After the second baby is delivered you will be given an injection of ergometrine in your thigh to ensure that the uterus contracts properly and to speed up the third stage—the birth of the placenta.

Pain relief in labor

FEW LABORS ARE PAINLESS but stories about suffering in labor are often exaggerated and distorted, and some women feel that severe pain is so inevitable that it becomes a self-fulfilling prophecy. The amount of pain actually felt almost always has a strong relationship to what is expected. Of course you should be realistic, but your expectations can be greatly modified by what you learn, the information you are given, and how confident you feel when you go into labor. This is why prenatal classes and breathing exercises, which give you the knowledge that you have some control over your body, and therefore some control over pain, are so important to you.

Everyone agrees that fear and ignorance cause tension, stress and anxiety, all of which make pain worse, and may even create pain where there is very little. Information, knowledge and support can go a long way to dispel fear and anxiety, and will also help to ease pain. There's no question that pain can be relieved with drugs, but to my mind the best form of pain relief is information, a calm state of mind and moral support. Armed with these you will find not only that the pain you feel is less, but that you may be strong enough to cope with it without resorting to analgesics or anesthetics which might dim your consciousness and awareness of what's going on—something that most women these days want to avoid.

Doctors and midwives believe that an important part of their job is to make labor as pain-free as possible and if they feel you are in difficulty they will be keen to offer you a range of analgesics. However, they will not force anything on you. It is a good idea to discuss pain relief at the prenatal clinic early in your pregnancy, to make your preferences clear (see p. 74) and have them recorded in your notes and birth plan (see p. 240). Remember to state alternatives in case things don't go according to plan.

Of course it's impossible to know your own pain threshold in advance and not all problems can be predicted. So it is important to go into labor with an open mind and to accept the pain relief offered if it is considered essential. Whatever happens, don't feel guilty; not everyone has a trouble-free labor and birth.

DECISION TO ACCEPT PAIN RELIEF

There are two important considerations about the use of painkilling drugs in labor. With most drugs, whether they're sedatives which make you feel calm and sleepy, hypnotics which actually send you to sleep, or narcotics which make you feel light-headed and cut off from the normal world, you will lose some awareness of what is happening around you. Many women want to experience every second of giving birth and any interference with their level of awareness is unacceptable. The second important factor is that most drugs will cross the placenta to the baby and will be in a higher concentration in the baby's blood than in the mother's blood. Many mothers find this unacceptable. Bearing both of these things in mind, and after getting as much information as you need, make up your mind about your attitude to having painkilling drugs in your labor.

A useful tip is to wait a little before accepting drugs. Some good news and moral support may be enough to get you over a sticky patch. Ask how far dilated you are. If you feel you are making good progress and can hang on, that may increase your resolve. Some encouraging words from your partner will give you added strength. So give yourself about 15 minutes after you feel you may want some pain relief before actually having it. During that time you may make quite good progress. You may even have got through the most painful parts of labor and have only a little way to go. You may be astonished at your own strength and resilience and feel that you can manage perfectly well without drugs.

ANALGESICS

Analgesics are drugs that relieve pain. They work by numbing the pain center of the brain. Inhalation analgesia (sometimes erroneously known as gas and air) is in fact a mixture of nitrous oxide and oxygen called Entonox. It is self-administered and you can inhale it half a minute before the peak of a contraction. You may become light-headed while inhaling it, but regain full consciousness a few seconds later. You might be given the opportunity to practice with the machine in your prenatal classes. Even if you don't use it successfully during labor, it gives you something to concentrate on while you are having contractions; this can be quite useful if you're becoming discouraged.

Pethidine is a narcotic given by injection in varying dosages during the first stage. It takes about 20 minutes to work and is sometimes combined with other drugs. Pethidine relaxes you and relieves your anxiety but its painkilling effect is variable. It is given less frequently than it used to be largely because it was used to relieve maternal fatigue if the first stage of labor was protracted. With modern aids, mothers no longer become overtired and distressed in the way they used to. The safest time to administer the drug is six to eight hours before delivery. As this is difficult to calculate and the drug wears off in about two hours, it is probably best for those women who are nervous and anxious during the early first stage of labor.

ENTONOX
Used properly, Entonox, also known as gas and air, gives a mild level of pain relief. The mask through which you breathe must fit firmly against your face.

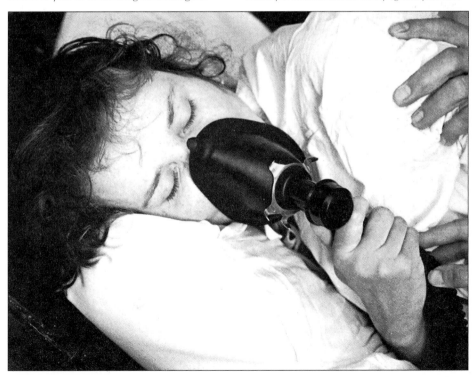

ANESTHETICS

A general anesthetic is never used during a normal birth, but a local or regional anesthetic may be given to dull your conscious appreciation of pain. Anesthetic is injected into a nerve root to numb the part of the body which the nerve supplies. The most widely used local anesthetic is the epidural (see right). In addition, before an episiotomy (see p. 198) and during stitching of the perineum after the birth (perineal infiltration) a pudendal block is administered, which numbs the lower part of the vagina by blocking the pudendal nerve.

EPIDURAL ANESTHESIA

The epidural, which has been called the Cadillac of anesthetics, prevents pain being felt in the abdominal area by acting as a "nerve block" in the spine. It probably has no effect on the fetus directly but it does affect you in labor. One of the reasons why the epidural has become so popular is that it fulfills all the criteria of a good pain reliever but in no way interferes with your awareness and your levels of consciousness. There are very few side effects associated with the majority of epidural anesthetics, and for many women it is a perfect answer.

HAVING AN EPIDURAL

An epidural takes about 10–20 minutes for a skilled anesthetist to set up. The analgesic effect is usually felt in just a few minutes and lasts for about two hours but you can be "topped up" when the pain returns and becomes severe.

SETTING UP AN EPIDURAL
You will be asked to lie on your left side, pulling your legs up to make as tight a ball as possible. Your lower back will be washed with cold spirit and then you will be given an injection of local anesthetic. A small hole will be made in your back with a solid needle and a hollow needle is then inserted in its place. Once the epidural space is located, a fine catheter is threaded through the hollow needle and into the epidural space, leaving a length of catheter protruding from your back. The catheter is secured to your skin along its length with paper tape. The local anesthetic is then given by syringe down the catheter and the opening is sealed. You will have a drip set up so that fluids can be fed to you intravenously should your blood pressure fall. A catheter will be inserted into your bladder to empty it.

THE POSITION FOR SETTING UP THE EPIDURAL

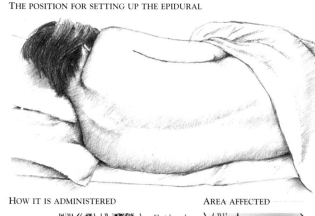

HOW IT IS ADMINISTERED

Hollow needle

Syringe

Catheter

AREA AFFECTED

Epidural space

Dura

Spinal cord

Vertebrae

HYPNOSIS

Hypnosis can relieve pain in a susceptible person. However, many practice sessions during pregnancy are advisable and both you and the hypnotist (see p. 244) should be familiar with what is required of you.

ACUPUNCTURE

I would recommend using acupuncture for pain relief in labor only if you have found it successful in the past. For some women it will undoubtedly work but the acupuncturist (see p. 245) must be practiced at giving pain relief in labor.

TENS

TENS stands for transcutaneous nerve stimulation and is a means of relieving labor pain by stimulating production of the body's natural painkillers—endorphins—and by blocking pain sensation with an electric current. The electrodes are placed on the woman's body and she is able to regulate the intensity of the current herself. TENS has been used successfully but it does not help everyone, particularly not those women who experience lots of pain. TENS doesn't relieve all of the pain but what remains is possibly easier to bear. A try-out before labor is advisable.

ADVANTAGES AND DISADVANTAGES OF AN EPIDURAL

ADVANTAGES

1 It provides complete pain relief without dulling any of your mental faculties.
2 It has a tendency to slow down labor, which can be useful.
3 No other local anesthetic will be necessary should you need forceps, vacuum extraction or episiotomy.
4 It allows you to participate in your birth if you have a cesarean, and the baby needs less resuscitation than with a general anesthetic.
5 As it lowers blood pressure it is ideal for women with pre-eclampsia or high blood pressure.
6 It can be topped up with extra anesthetic or allowed to wear off near the delivery so that you can control the actual birth. The contractions at this stage may be a bit of a shock, though, if you haven't experienced any until then.
7 It reduces the amount of work done by the lungs in labor and so can benefit women with heart or lung disease.
8 It reduces muscular activity in the legs and is therefore of value to diabetic women, making their insulin and glucose requirements easier to balance.

DISADVANTAGES

1 Makes for a medically managed birth from the start. A skilled anesthetist must be present.
2 The lowering of blood pressure may make you feel dizzy and nauseous. This is more likely if you lie on your back so turn onto your side.
3 There is the possibility of a post-anesthetic headache which lasts a few hours after delivery.
4 There is a possibility of an episiotomy and a forceps delivery. Depending on the concentration of the anesthetic, there may be a loss of muscle power and of the sensation of the contractions. This results in a slower second stage because you will be entirely dependent on the instructions of the midwife as to when to push the baby out. The length of the second stage is the factor that determines the use of forceps.
5 If the mother's blood pressure drops, the amount of blood supplying the placenta is reduced and so the oxygen supply to the baby is lowered.
6 If it is allowed to wear off, the contractions may come as a nasty shock.
7 Not all epidurals are effective.

PAIN RELIEF IN LABOR

TYPE OF DRUG	ACTION	EFFECT ON MOTHER & BABY
NARCOTICS (morphine, pethidine)	Sedate and relieve anxiety. Possibly relieve pain during the first stage of labor.	Reduce consciousness and tend to make the labor longer. Cross the placenta in five minutes and can depress respiration at birth. Sucking may be inefficient (see p. 215). Can produce nausea in the mother.
INHALATION ANALGESIA (Entonox)	Relieves pain. Can cause drowsiness if allowed to accumulate.	Depresses alertness but this returns once the effects have worn off. Makes you lightheaded while breathing in the gas. No significant effect on the baby.

Medical intervention

DURING THE LAST 20 years hospital childbirth has been revolutionized by the development of new procedures which have been widely adopted as routine practice. All offer advantages; a few carry risks, though small. None of them should be used unless there are good medical reasons. Most people believe that the convenience of the staff or even of the mother should not be the sole justification for the employment of these procedures.

EPISIOTOMY

In an episiotomy, which takes place during the second stage of labor, an incision is made in the perineum between the vaginal opening and the anus to facilitate delivery of the baby. It is the most common operation in the western world.

The cut is made with scissors under a local anesthetic just as the baby's head appears. If it is done too early, before the perineum has thinned out, muscles, skin and blood vessels are damaged and the bleeding may be profuse. Also the tissues are crushed by the scissors as they are cut. This leads to bruising, swelling and slow healing and accounts for a great deal of

the pain and discomfort which often follows episiotomy. There is also the possibility that the integrity of the pelvic floor can be damaged if the muscle fibers are not correctly aligned. If the vagina and perineum are stitched too tightly a woman may experience discomfort when intercourse is resumed. You might like to

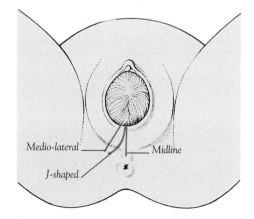

EPISIOTOMY INCISIONS
The different types of incision include the medio-lateral, from the back of the vagina out to the side; the midline, which runs between the vagina and the anus; and the J-shaped cut, which combines the two.

have it recorded in your notes that you wish to avoid having an episiotomy if it is at all possible.

There are grounds for suspecting that episiotomy may have become an obstetric fashion. If medical staff indicate that they think an episiotomy is necessary during labor, you should ask why it's being done.

AVOIDING AN EPISIOTOMY

One of the best ways to avoid the necessity for an episiotomy is to deliver your baby in as upright a position as you possibly can (see p. 64). Tell your midwife early in labor that you want to find a good position for the second stage of labor and in particular that you'd like to avoid lying on your back. Together with your birth partner, your midwife will then be ready to help give you the support you need when the time comes.

If you learn how to relax the muscles of the pelvic floor prenatally and allow your vaginal tissues and perineum to bulge out (see p. 125) you can avoid a tear. Familiarity with the sensation when the baby's head bulges or "crowns" will mean that you will realize that you are starting to tighten up in the second stage and you can try to do something about it.

REASONS FOR AN EPISIOTOMY

An episiotomy will be necessary if:
● The perineum hasn't had time to stretch slowly—breathing exercises and massage help with this.
● The baby's head is too large for the vaginal opening.
● You aren't able to control your pushing so that you can stop when necessary and then push gradually and smoothly. An episiotomy will deliver the baby quickly if you have difficulty with coordination and control of pushing in the second stage.
● The baby is distressed.
● You have a forceps or ventouse (vacuum extraction) delivery.
● Yours is a breech birth.

Having an epidural anesthetic may increase the possibility of having an episiotomy. If you do opt for an epidural, there is no reason why an episiotomy is automatically necessary but you will need to make your views known and try to have the end of the second stage well under your control by relaxing the pelvic floor muscle and not pushing down too hard when the head is delivered. I had an epidural twice but on neither occasion did I have an episiotomy.

EXPERIENCE OF EPISIOTOMY

Sheila Kitzinger, in her study of 2000 women who had episiotomies, came to the following conclusions:
● Episiotomies were more painful than a tear.
● Women found it more difficult to get into a comfortable position to hold the baby after an episiotomy.
● The pain distracted them during breastfeeding.
● An episiotomy was more likely to give pain or discomfort during sexual intercourse even three months after delivery.
● Two-thirds of the women had never discussed episiotomy with medical staff during pregnancy. Some had tried but had been unsuccessful.
● About half the episiotomies had been done when the perineum was not sufficiently thinned out.
● More than half the women had not been instructed to release the vagina and pelvic floor muscles but had been encouraged to push instead, which made the episiotomy more necessary.
● About one-quarter of the women had not been told to stop pushing while the head was being born to give the vagina a chance to thin out.
● More than a third of the women were never given a reason for the episiotomy.
● Some women found the stitching painful but when they complained they were told (incorrectly) that there were no nerve endings there.

INDUCTION

Induction is the artificial "starting off" of labor. Your labor will be induced should it fail to start on its own or if for some reason your doctor decides that you need to deliver the baby early.

Induction is usually planned in advance; depending on the hospital, you may be admitted the night before or you may simply come into the hospital on the day. Induction is often introduced gradually, first with prostaglandin suppositories, then if necessary, by rupturing the membranes (ARM), and finally, if things are going too slowly, with an oxytocin drip.

PROSTAGLANDIN SUPPOSITORIES

No one knows exactly why labor starts but suppositories or a gel containing prostaglandins, which are made up of various hormones that have an effect on a pregnant woman's uterus, are used to induce labor.

The use of prostaglandin suppositories is the least invasive method of starting labor. Suppositories are inserted into the vagina, and labor will usually start within a few hours. Sometimes a single suppository may be enough, but more than one may be needed to get things going. In 50 percent of cases the prostaglandin suppositories may be supplemented with ARM and an oxytocin drip.

ARTIFICIAL RUPTURE OF THE MEMBRANES

Also known as ARM or amniotomy, rupturing the membranes is only done if the cervix is sufficiently open and the head is low in the pelvis. It doesn't in itself stimulate contractions although they may start spontaneously. However, ARM often needs supplementing with oxytocin to stimulate contractions, because labor must begin within 24 hours to avoid the risk of infection.

A pair of forceps or a tool not unlike a crochet hook is inserted into the womb and a small opening is made in the membrane so that the waters escape. For most women this is a painless procedure. Labor usually reaches full intensity quickly after ARM because the baby's head is no longer cushioned and presses hard against the cervix, encouraging the uterus to contract.

Amniotomy was until fairly recently almost a routine procedure during the preparation for any labor. If left alone, the waters don't usually break until late in the first stage of labor. There are two major disadvantages of amniotomy. The first is that it makes the labor proceed more quickly and intensely than it would normally. Also, if the baby has the cord around its neck, the loss of fluid increases pressure and can affect the flow of blood through the cord to the baby.

AMNIOTOMY
The bag of waters usually ruptures naturally towards the end of the first stage of labor. Before it breaks, it provides a cushion for the baby's head as it presses against the cervix (right). Once the membranes have ruptured (far right), the contractions increase in intensity because the baby's head is now resting hard against the cervix. This speeds up labor, which is why amniotomy may be performed if progress is slow.

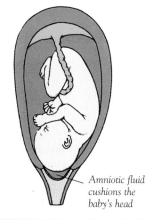

Amniotic fluid cushions the baby's head

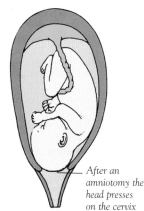

After an amniotomy the head presses on the cervix

Besides being a method of induction, amniotomy will be performed if an electrode is to be attached to the baby's head to monitor its heartbeat (see p. 202); if the baby's heart rate goes down, the amniotic fluid can be examined for traces of meconium, the first bowel movements of the baby. Meconium in the fluid can indicate fetal distress.

OXYTOCIN-INDUCED LABOR

The hormone oxytocin, which is produced by the pituitary gland in the brain, stimulates the uterus to start contracting. It is therefore given in a synthetic form to start labor off and to keep it going.

Oxytocin is normally given via a drip inserted into a vein. Ask for it to be inserted in the arm you use least and check that you have a long tube connecting you to the drip. You should then have more room to move around, even if just on the bed. The drip can be turned down if you go into strong labor quickly and the cervix becomes half dilated. The needle won't be removed from your arm until after the baby is born as the uterus needs to keep contracting to expel the placenta and then prevent bleeding (see p. 190).

The contractions you experience while on an oxytocin drip are often stronger, longer and more painful, with shorter periods of relaxation in between. Unfortunately this may mean the need for painkilling drugs is greater. Also, the blood supply to the uterus is temporarily shut off during each strong contraction, which may be detrimental to the baby.

REASONS FOR INDUCTION

Forty years ago induction was frequently used for hospital or social convenience. Induction was sometimes planned to suit working hours or changes in shifts, for example. In the sixties and seventies, obstetrics went through a phase of over-zealous high-tech intervention, when there

was a great vogue for induced labors, especially in older mothers who, at that time, were much less common than today. Oxytocin-induced labor was once used in as many as 40–50 percent of deliveries. Given that the rate of success with this form of induction is only about 85 percent, its routine use cannot be justified, and most modern obstetricians believe that less than a few percent of pregnant women require it. Nowadays fewer than one in five labors are induced by any method and I'd like to reassure you that induction is a great asset provided it's done strictly for medical reasons, such as pre-eclampsia.

Only five percent of babies actually come on the due date and it's hard for some doctors and quite a lot of mothers to remain philosophical when that magic date passes. Both are concerned in case the baby is "postmature," or late. The fear is that the placenta may be becoming inadequate to support the baby and the baby is outgrowing its food supply.

Very few babies are truly overdue, however; 80 percent of all babies who are born with a spontaneous labor arrive after the due date. This is mainly because medical convention calculates the expected date of delivery from the last menstrual period rather than from the time of conception (see p. 49). Most doctors accept that up to 14 days after the expected date of delivery is normal and won't suggest intervening before then unless maternal or fetal health is giving cause for concern. After 14 days, signs of postmaturity are carefully looked for. Screening involves monitoring the fetal heart and movements and ultrasound for amniotic fluid measurement.

However, waiting until the expected day of delivery is leaving it a bit late to face the prospect of an induced labor. This is something that should be read about and discussed earlier on in pregnancy and you and your doctor should try to agree on the course to be followed should induction be necessary in your case.

ELECTRONIC FETAL MONITORING

Electronic fetal monitoring (EFM) is a method of recording the baby's heartbeat and your contractions during labor. It is the high-tech replacement for the ear trumpet or fetoscope, but has by no means superseded these. Almost all maternity units ask you to be monitored routinely for about 20 minutes, but if all is well there is no need for you to be continuously monitored.

Monitoring is usually done with belts strapped around your abdomen that simultaneously pick up contractions and the baby's heartbeat, recording them on a graph. The print-out can then be interpreted by the midwife to make sure that the baby's heart is beating normally during the contraction (see below right). During a contraction blood flow to your placenta is reduced for a few seconds and your baby's heart rate dips. It then returns to normal when the contraction passes. Occasionally doctors may think it necessary to attach an electrode to the baby's scalp as well, if the

MONITORING IN LABOR

Many women find the monitor reassuring. They can see the contractions coming and prepare for them and they can watch their baby's heartbeat throughout labor.

FETAL MONITOR ELECTRODE

If your medical team think that your baby needs closer monitoring, they may want to attach an electrode to his head. Once your cervix is at least 2–3 centimeters dilated, you will be given an amniotomy to break your waters (see p. 200) if they haven't broken already. An electrode is then attached to the part of the baby that is going to be born first, which is usually his head. The electrode pierces the skin slightly and provides an electrical contact that tracks the baby's heartbeat. Electronic signals are then relayed to the external monitor and a graph is printed out for the staff to interpret.

abdominal recording is of poor quality and your baby is thought to need constant monitoring. The electrode is attached to his presenting part, usually to the skin on the top of his head, and picks up his heartbeat. It is an accurate method of monitoring, but it does mean that your waters will have to be broken if they haven't already done so.

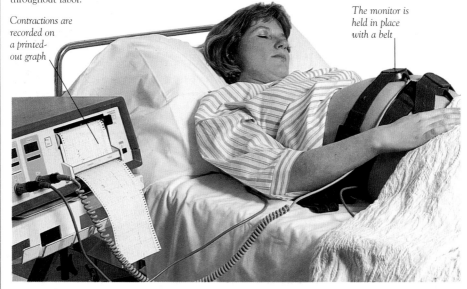

Contractions are recorded on a printed-out graph

The monitor is held in place with a belt

CONTINUOUS EFM

Monitoring the baby's heartbeat and the uterine contractions is essential if you are being induced (see p. 200), if your labor is being accelerated or if you have an epidural, when you will be less able to feel the onset of contractions. Most hospitals now agree that EFM should be used routinely in high-risk pregnancies.

Electronic fetal monitoring involving a fetal scalp electrode used to confine mothers to bed but nowadays it is less restricting. A method of monitoring by radio waves, known as telemetry, allows the mother to walk about away from the monitoring equipment. The electrode is still attached to the baby's head but it is joined to a strap on the mother's thigh and not to a large machine. However, babies do suffer rashes where the electrode was clipped to them and there is no proof that they feel no pain. Electronic fetal monitoring provides the medical staff with a second-by-second report

PROBLEMS WITH CONTINUOUS EFM

- The staff are more aware of any small changes and may therefore be more likely to intervene rather than letting labor take its natural course.
- Babies who are electronically monitored are three times more likely to be delivered by cesarean section.
- EFM increases the electronic paraphernalia in the delivery room.
- Staff may be tempted to concentrate more on the machine than on the woman in labor.
- EFM may restrict movement, thus slowing down the labor and making fetal distress more likely.
- Attaching the electrode may bruise and hurt the baby's head.

on the condition of your baby, so that they can intervene quickly if he is in distress. If a doctor tells you that you need continuous EFM, try to see that as reassuring, because it will ensure that you get the best possible care for your baby.

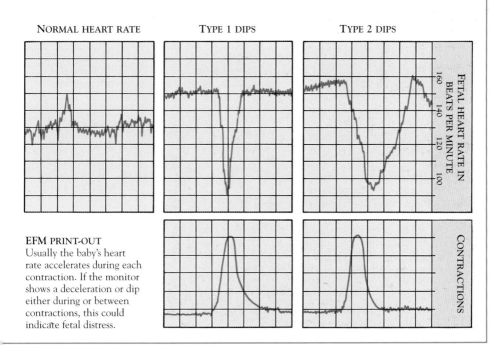

| NORMAL HEART RATE | TYPE 1 DIPS | TYPE 2 DIPS |

FETAL HEART RATE IN BEATS PER MINUTE

CONTRACTIONS

EFM PRINT-OUT
Usually the baby's heart rate accelerates during each contraction. If the monitor shows a deceleration or dip either during or between contractions, this could indicate fetal distress.

16
Complications of the birth

E ven the best planned labors may not go according to plan, especially for first-time mothers. You may become exhausted or your baby may become distressed and need to be delivered quickly. Thinking about the possibility of a cesarean or forceps delivery in advance will help you to know what to expect should the situation arise.

Breech birth

A BREECH BABY is one that is born buttocks first. Most babies are in the breech position until about the 32nd week of pregnancy when they turn head down (cephalic position). Four out of every hundred babies, however, stay put. If your baby is one of these, do not be concerned; most breech labors are smooth, though you will have to have the baby in a hospital. Doctors used to try to turn breech babies by applying gentle external pressure on the abdomen. This procedure is rarely performed now.

Doctors do not generally recommend a home birth if the baby is in the breech position. However, if you are at home, try to adopt a supported upright position with your legs wide apart and your knees bent to give the baby's head more space.

After the birth, your genital region might be slightly swollen but the swelling will subside within 48 hours. Because many breech births are helped by forceps, babies may have bruises on the face and head, but they will fade fast. You are more likely to have an episiotomy (see p. 198)

with a breech birth because the head has less time to be compressed during delivery, making it more likely to get stuck.

Attitudes towards breech births differ: some doctors feel that a breech baby should always be delivered by cesarean section, others are less rigid. However, about 80 percent of breech babies are delivered by cesarean section in the US.

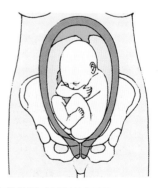

A WELL-FLEXED BREECH BABY
It is possible to deliver a baby in this position vaginally, though an episiotomy may be necessary.

BIRTH OF A BREECH BABY

The baby's buttocks press against the cervix and effacement and dilatation of the cervix occur as with a cephalic presentation (see p. 176). The waters usually break early with a breech presentation and you will probably feel contractions as bad backache (see p. 181). Kneeling on all fours is a helpful position to relieve this during the first stage. For the birth, the supported squatting position is safest and an episiotomy may be done in this position if necessary, though your doctor may prefer the lithotomy position (see p. 64). Sometimes forceps may be used to protect the baby's head during delivery and therefore epidurals are increasingly being given for breech births. If you then need a cesarean section, this will save time and allow you to hold your baby the moment he is born.

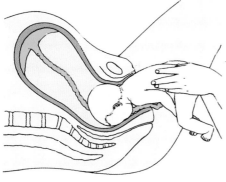

DELIVERING THE BODY
The buttocks are delivered first and then the legs. While the body is being delivered, it is better to breathe through the contractions than to push. Before the head is delivered you may be given an episiotomy, and forceps are inserted at this point.

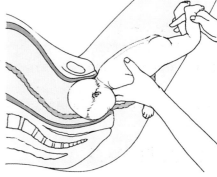

DELIVERING THE HEAD
The weight of the baby's body draws the head down to the vagina and the body is then lifted to deliver the head. Doctors usually use forceps to protect the head from too much compression, and one push is usually enough to deliver the baby.

Cesarean section

INEVITABLY THERE ARE slight risks associated with cesarean section, as it is a major operation. There is the risk attached to having a general anesthetic and the risk of bleeding or clot formation which is always possible with major surgery; there is also the disadvantage of being left with a scar on the uterus that may weaken it. The rate of cesarean sections is still rising so there is some concern that the operation is undertaken without enough thought.

You may know weeks or only days in advance that you are to have your baby by cesarean section. This is known as a planned or "elective" cesarean. You will be admitted to a hospital on a certain day, but if you go into labor spontaneously beforehand, you will still be given a cesarean. Some cesareans are performed as emergencies when it's essential that the baby is delivered quickly. Cesareans can be done under an epidural or spinal anesthetic (see p. 196), which is safer for you and the baby and means you can be conscious throughout. However, if an epidural isn't already in place at the time, an emergency cesarean would have to be done under general anesthetic.

PREPARING FOR A CESAREAN

Some women find a cesarean section a great disappointment after looking forward to a vaginal delivery, especially if the hospital unit is not one that allows mothers and fathers to participate actively in the cesarean labor and birth, and have immediate and intimate contact with the baby at birth and afterwards. Some women feel guilty that they've let their partner down and that he couldn't be there with them at the time of birth. Many mothers are angered and disappointed if they're not able to have their baby with them after the operation and have to be separated just at the time when mother and baby need each other for mutual support. But these psychological effects can be minimized if you prepare yourself for having a cesarean section and look on it as a positive experience.

Ask to see your obstetrician so that you and your partner can have a relaxed discussion about what the operation entails, what the procedures will be in the operating room, whether you can have epidural anesthesia and be awake and alert during the operation and whether your partner can be with you.

Ask your hospital clinic if there is a video available that shows what happens during a cesarean. You can also prepare yourself by talking to other women who have had cesarean sections. This is one of the best ways of preventing you from having negative feelings about it. Not only will you get moral support but you'll also get useful information about what it feels like, how long it takes to be completely fit again after the operation and tips on caring for your baby while your wound is healing. By talking to mothers who've had subsequent pregnancies after a cesarean section, you can allay your fears about the future. A self-help group will be able to put you in touch with midwives and obstetricians who have a flexible and realistic attitude to pregnancy after cesarean section.

WHAT HAPPENS

Your pubic hair will be shaved, the epidural anesthesia will be set up, you'll have an intravenous drip inserted into your arm so that fluids can be fed directly into your bloodstream, and a catheter will be inserted into your bladder to drain away urine. A screen will probably be placed in front of your face and your partner might prefer to stand behind it at your head if he doesn't want to see the surgical procedure. A cesarean section usually takes about 45 minutes but the baby is delivered within the first 5–10 minutes. The remaining time is for stitching the uterine wall and the abdomen. A small horizontal incision is made (see below) and the amniotic fluid is then drained off by suction—you'll hear this quite clearly. The baby is then gently lifted out either by hand or with forceps. You will be given an injection of ergometrine to make the uterus contract and to prevent bleeding. You and your partner can hold the baby while the third stage is completed. If everything is all right you can start nursing him as soon as possible. Depending on the reasons for the operation, your baby may be taken away to special care for an observation period. The catheter and the drip will remain in for some hours and the stitches or clamps will be removed five days later.

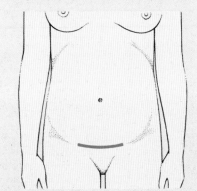

THE HORIZONTAL LINE INCISION
The so-called "bikini line" incision is common for obvious cosmetic reasons and because the low transverse cut heals more effectively.

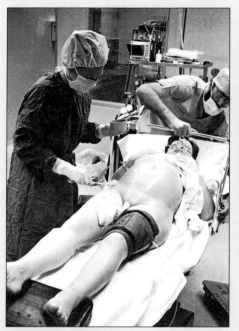

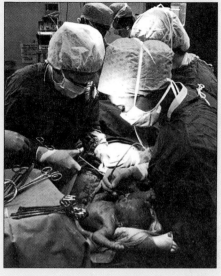

HAVING A CESAREAN
Once the epidural is set up and you are prepared for surgery, the baby's birth is very quick. Your partner can hold the baby while you are stitched.

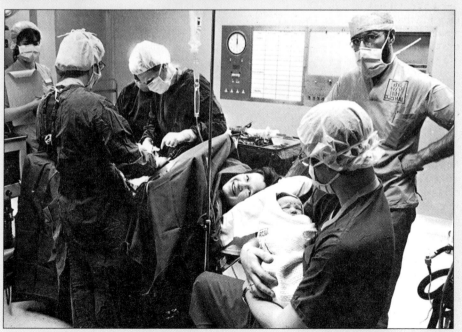

RETURNING TO NORMAL

After the operation you will return to the postnatal ward with your baby. Because you need plenty of rest after abdominal surgery, you can concentrate on feeding the baby and getting to know him. You will be expected to get up and move around the next day and you can start gentle exercises (see p. 228)

after two days. Most mothers feel normal from one week onwards after the operation. You will lose blood from the vagina just as you would after a vaginal delivery. You must take care when lifting and avoid strenuous activity for at least six weeks. The scar will fade, usually in 3–6 months.

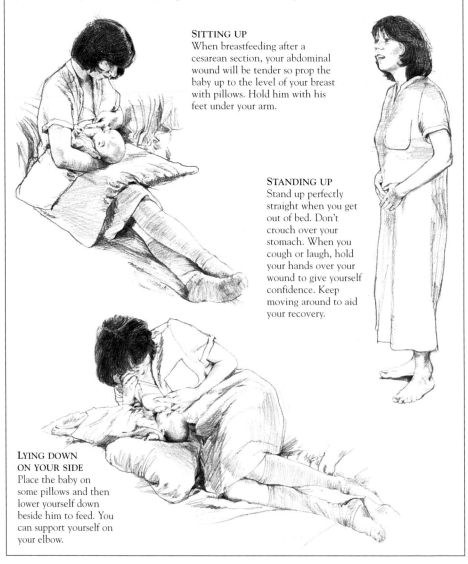

SITTING UP
When breastfeeding after a cesarean section, your abdominal wound will be tender so prop the baby up to the level of your breast with pillows. Hold him with his feet under your arm.

STANDING UP
Stand up perfectly straight when you get out of bed. Don't crouch over your stomach. When you cough or laugh, hold your hands over your wound to give yourself confidence. Keep moving around to aid your recovery.

LYING DOWN ON YOUR SIDE
Place the baby on some pillows and then lower yourself down beside him to feed. You can support yourself on your elbow.

REASONS FOR A CESAREAN SECTION

- Prolapse of the umbilical cord through the cervix.
- Placenta previa (see p. 156).
- Abruptio placentae (see p. 156).
- Fetus shows signs of profound distress; this will be obvious if the heart rate slows or "dips" at each contraction and, more seriously, between each contraction—this will show up on the print-out from the electronic monitors (see p. 202). If there is meconium in the amniotic fluid, the baby may have had a bowel movement which could indicate distress.
- The baby needs to be delivered early and induction and labor are considered to be an unnecessary risk to the baby or the mother.
- The baby is extremely large or there may be cephalo-pelvic disproportion, where the baby's head is larger than the pelvic cavity.
- Breech babies (see p. 204) are often delivered by cesarean section, particularly in the United States.
- A previous baby was born by this method; this is the commonest reason for the operation in the United States.
- A serious infection of the vagina, such as a first-time attack of genital herpes.
- The cervix fails to dilate.
- Forceps fail to deliver the baby.
- Serious Rhesus incompatibility.

Some of the conditions that warrant abdominal delivery of the baby may not be apparent until labor has begun, and this will then result in an emergency cesarean section. Unless you already had an epidural in place and depending on the reasons for the emergency cesarean, you will be given a general anesthetic, although a good alternative is a spinal anesthetic (which is like an epidural but cannot be topped up).

Forceps delivery

ONE OF THE ARGUMENTS put forward by the advocates of natural childbirth is that forceps are being commonly required because mothers are routinely given drugs and anesthetics that interfere with their own efforts to deliver the baby. In other words, a certain proportion of forceps deliveries are probably doctor induced. For centuries obstetric forceps offered the only method of delivery that was not a natural one. As cesarean section has become safer, the use of forceps has declined, so that they are no longer used for any hazardous type of delivery. Nowadays, forceps are applied only when the first stage is complete, the cervix is fully dilated and the baby's head has descended well into the mother's pelvis but has failed to descend any further, or there are signs of either fetal or maternal distress.

A forceps delivery is normally done with the mother in the lithotomy position (see p. 64). Your legs will be put into stirrups

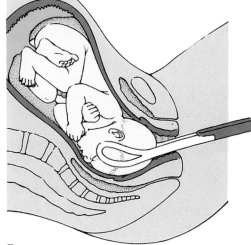

FORCEPS
Designed to fit snugly over the baby's head, forceps are rather like a cage protecting the baby's head from any pressure in the birth canal. They may cause a little bruising but this soon fades.

and a local anesthetic will be injected into the perineum. The forceps, which are shaped rather like serving tongs, are inserted into your vagina one side at a time. The doctor will have already determined where the baby's head lies and with gentle pulling on the forceps for 30–40 seconds at a time, and in time with your contractions, the baby's head gradually descends to the perineum.

There should be little pain. An episiotomy (see p. 198) is then performed. When the head is delivered, the forceps are removed and the delivery can be completed normally.

If longer forceps are needed to pull the baby out, you may be given a pudendal nerve block, which is a local anesthetic that is injected into the vaginal wall (see p. 196).

Jaundice

JAUNDICE IS FAIRLY COMMON in newborn babies around about the third day of life. Medically it's called physiological jaundice, which means that it has no sinister connotations. A baby is born with a large number of red blood cells, which are rapidly broken down after it is born. When red blood cells break down and are replaced, they release large quantities of the pigment known as bilirubin, which gives them their color, and this has to be removed by the liver. At the time of birth a baby's liver is still immature and is not able to carry the excess load of bilirubin so the levels of

pigments rise in the blood and give the skin a yellowish tinge. This type of jaundice usually fades at the end of the first week when the liver has cleared the blood of pigment. The baby may be rather sleepy.

To help flush the excess bilirubin out of the baby's system, feed him often—you may have wake him to feed. If bilirubin levels are high, the baby may be given light treatment (phototherapy). The baby's eyes are covered and he is placed naked in a crib under an ultraviolet light. The light breaks down the bilirubin so that it can be passed more quickly by the baby in urine.

Postpartum hemorrhage

BLEEDING AFTER THE BIRTH is rare largely because the uterus has a self-protecting device to stop it from bleeding. Once the fetus and the placenta have been expelled and the uterus is completely empty, it usually contracts down rapidly to about the size of a tennis ball. This contraction closes the uterine arteries so that they cannot bleed. Under normal circumstances therefore, little bleeding occurs after the delivery and there is little chance of infection. A uterus that is not empty, however, is not able to contract down tightly enough to arrest bleeding from the uterine arteries, and occasionally the uterus

doesn't contract properly even though it is empty. In either case, this bleeding is called postpartum hemorrhage. The commonest cause of postpartum bleeding is a small fragment of placenta left in the uterus, usually diagnosed by examining the placenta and finding that a portion is missing. Under these circumstances, the mother is informed of what is going on, is anesthetized and the placenta is gently scraped away from inside the uterus.

If bleeding occurs more than 24 hours after delivery, the lochia (see p. 219) may become bright red again. This can occur as a result of overexerting yourself. Your doctor will probably advise you to rest for several days. If the bleeding recurs or becomes heavy, this can mean infection or the retention of a small piece of placenta. Your doctor will probably prescribe antibiotics to cure the problem. If not, she may refer you back to the hospital. If you pass clots, call an ambulance to take you to the nearest accident and emergency unit where the inner surface of your womb will be thoroughly but gently cleansed.

Prematurity

A BABY THAT IS BORN at less than 37 completed weeks of pregnancy is said to be premature, regardless of birthweight. A baby that weighs less than 5 lb (2.5 kg) at term has a low birthweight. Either of these situations may involve a baby in some form of special care after birth. The cause of prematurity remains a mystery in about 40 percent of cases, but various factors that predispose are pre-eclampsia (see p. 162), multiple pregnancy (see p. 159), premature rupture of the membranes and abnormal placenta. Some maternal diseases, such as anemia or malnutrition, and overwork, can also have an effect.

Fibroids and sometimes an ovarian cyst may be an underlying cause.

As a general rule, a premature labor begins without any warning and the first sign may be rupture of the membranes, the beginning of uterine contractions or some vaginal bleeding. Provided it isn't too far advanced, attempts may be made to stop a premature labor so that the mother can be given steroid injections to mature the fetal lungs and to reduce the

GETTING TO KNOW YOUR PREMATURE BABY
Parents are encouraged to touch and care for their babies in the special care baby unit.

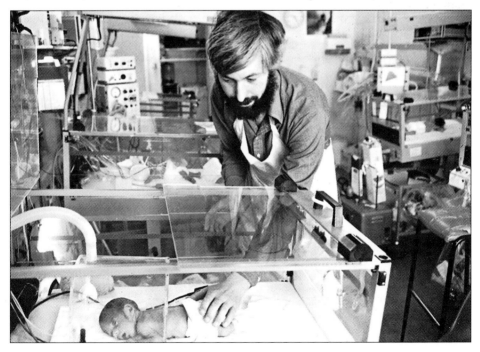

work of breathing after the birth. This means the mother must be admitted to the hospital and monitored closely. Usually a premature labor is shorter and easier than a full-term labor, mainly because the head of the baby, the largest part, is smaller and softer than that of a full-term baby. Nearly all premature births therefore are accompanied by an episiotomy in order to protect the baby's soft head from pressure changes inside the birth canal.

The three most important aspects of a premature baby's health are his ability to breathe, feed and control his temperature. For these reasons the baby is nursed in a sterile incubator where the temperature is controlled, where the oxygen supply can be easily changed according to the baby's needs, and where feeding can be achieved by a tube passed down the baby's nose. Because he will have poor resistance to infection, care is taken to keep equipment sterile and you'll be shown by the staff how to handle your baby safely.

If you are afraid that bonding may not take place, be reassured. Parents are encouraged to feed, touch and nurse their baby as soon as his condition allows, but until that time they're encouraged to watch the nurses caring for their baby. Breast milk can be particularly valuable for a premature baby, so you can use a pump to provide breast milk for your baby and to establish your milk supply so that it is ready for him when he can suck on his own. A very premature baby (24–30 weeks), however, may initially be fed intravenously with a special solution.

Stillbirth

A BABY IS STILLBORN very rarely—it happens in fewer than one per hundred births. If the baby dies in the uterus before the 24th week the uterus usually goes spontaneously into labor within a day or so and a miscarriage will result. After 24 weeks the uterus will deliver the baby fairly quickly. Most, though not all, women are aware that something is wrong, usually because they have not felt any movements for 24 hours or more.

No one knows quite why a baby should die in late pregnancy, but in most cases it is thought to be due to an insufficiently healthy placenta. The placenta may have failed to grow adequately or have become diseased in some way during the pregnancy so that it is no longer able to maintain an adequate oxygen and food supply to the baby. Occasionally the placenta begins to separate from the uterus and this can cause intrauterine death. Uncontrolled Rhesus disease (see p. 162) or poorly stabilized diabetes can also lead to a stillbirth. When the baby dies, most of the sensations of being pregnant fade quite quickly as the levels of estrogen and progesterone plummet. Even the uterus may diminish in size due to the absorption of the amniotic fluid from around the fetus. This may show up in the mother as dramatic weight loss, which is always taken seriously at a prenatal check. If a baby's death is suspected, an ultrasonic scan will be done to try to detect the fetal heartbeat. If the heart cannot be detected by the scan, it's unlikely that the baby is still alive.

Because the baby is in a kind of cocoon inside the mother's body, its death does not adversely affect the mother's physical health. However, the emotional and psychological effects on both parents can be extremely traumatic. A woman will quite naturally feel all kinds of guilt, inadequacy, self-loathing, sadness and depression, and she may feel that she wants to withdraw and be completely by herself to come to terms with her grief. This can drive a wedge between her and her partner. You both need as much support as possible at this time, so for your own sakes, talk to each other about your feelings and talk to sympathetic friends and your doctor. It is also a good idea to seek bereavement counseling so that you can grieve fully and finally come to terms with your loss. Don't be surprised if this takes some time, even several months, but look forward to the future; most couples who have lost a baby do eventually become proud parents of healthy babies.

Until recently it was always thought that labor should be allowed to start spontaneously—it usually begins within two or three days of the baby's death—and should not be interfered with. However, most women find that they want to deliver the baby as soon as possible after its death has been confirmed, and in any case, labor is induced quickly to avoid the possibility of infection. Delivery of a stillborn baby by cesarean section is not recommended as it can increase the risk of infection, but there are no barriers to pain relief for a woman in this situation.

Many parents who have experienced a stillbirth find that touching, holding and naming their baby help them to come to terms with the loss. It also helps to have a photograph of the baby and to hold a proper funeral to say goodbye. The hospital will help you with the arrangements if you wish or you can make your own with a local funeral director. Ask your doctor to explain the reasons for your loss, but accept that no one may know exactly why your baby died. You may find that it helps to get in touch with others who have suffered this disappointment (see p. 244)—their experience can help you to understand your own reactions.

Vacuum extraction (ventouse)

VACUUM EXTRACTION MAY BE USED as an alternative to a forceps delivery, except where the mother is unable to push. It is used when there is a delay in the second stage of labor but where an easy delivery is ultimately anticipated. The head does not have to be in the birth canal, unlike for a forceps delivery.

The cervix is usually almost fully dilated for this procedure, which is sometimes known as ventouse extraction. A small metal or rubber cup connected to a vacuum apparatus is passed into the vagina and applied to the baby's head. It takes less than five minutes to put in place. When a vacuum has been created, the cup sticks to the baby's scalp, and by gentle pulling, and the mother pushing with her contractions, the baby's head is brought down into the pelvis and then slowly and gradually delivered.

There are few serious complications associated with vacuum extraction and there is much less potential for damage to the mother with vacuum extraction than with forceps. There may be a slight swelling on the baby's head where the metal cup applied suction, although this usually settles down within a day or so of delivery.

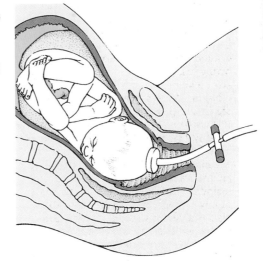

THE VACUUM EXTRACTOR
A form of birth assistance, the vacuum extractor is mainly used in Europe; forceps are favored in the U.S.

17

The first days

The birth of your baby is a climax to the nine months of waiting and anything that follows must, to a certain extent, fall in its shadow. During the first three days while you're waiting for the milk to come in, you may feel excited or tentative or you may find yourself in a state of shock. It's thrilling to explore your new baby and to enjoy quiet moments together, but don't be surprised if at times it feels like a bit of a letdown.

If you are in the hospital for a few days after the birth, it's important to look and learn from the midwives and the experienced mothers on the ward. However, if you're a first-time mother, don't compare yourself with them and don't resent their experienced handling of their babies. The most important advice I can give you is to be easy on yourself. Don't try to be the perfect mother, and don't try to accomplish too much in these first days. You should remember to take one day at a time.

Bonding

IT'S DIFFICULT TO DESCRIBE what bonding is; it's certainly getting to know your baby and exploring her with your eyes, nose, ears, fingertips and mouth, and even your tongue. It's also to do with attachment, protectiveness and possessiveness. This early attachment is possibly the strongest bond between human beings, and necessarily so, as it ensures the nurturing of infants, and hence the survival of the human race.

Establishing a relationship with your baby begins the second she is born. If possible you should be left in private with your partner with a minimum of interruption for some time during the first hour after the birth. Research has shown that babies are usually quiet but very alert in the first hour of life, and in this state they are extremely responsive. They will stare intently at your face if held 8–10 in. (20–25 cm) away. They can focus their eyes at this distance and respond to the human face. In addition, like most newborn animals, human babies have an instinct to bond with their parents. This is the right time for attachment to a caring adult, so both of you should make the most of it. Keep the lighting low and lay your baby against your body so that you make skin-to-skin contact. Looking into your baby's eyes renders her a person and not a thing, and skin contact allows you to feel each other as warm human beings.

The midwife may want to stitch you at this time, because early stitching is quicker and easier than if left until later, when the tissues may be swollen. It will probably be possible to hold your baby while it is being done or else your partner can have valuable one-to-one contact with his new baby. Other cleaning up can wait awhile.

All aspects of the bonding process—your voice, smell, touch, caresses, fondling—are good for the baby, and they're also good for you. The sooner you touch and fondle your baby, the more quickly your bleeding will cease, the more strongly your uterus will contract and the better your breasts will respond with the letdown of colostrum (see p. 221) and later milk. You are also increasing your confidence in handling the baby and helping her adapt to a new environment. Studies show that babies adapt more easily when they are held, soothed, crooned at and allowed to feed at will. Soon after you take hold of your baby, try putting her to your breast. Touch her cheek with your nipple and she will turn towards the breast. If she shows little perseverance—she may be sleepy if you had drugs for pain relief—express a little colostrum onto her lips to encourage her. Your partner can help by supporting the baby's head until you feel comfortable.

You may not bond instantly, however, particularly if you had a long or difficult labor. Don't worry; you have plenty of time to get to know your baby later.

THE FIRST HOUR OF LIFE
Your baby is very alert during the first hour after a normal birth so try to make the most of this precious time to get to know her.

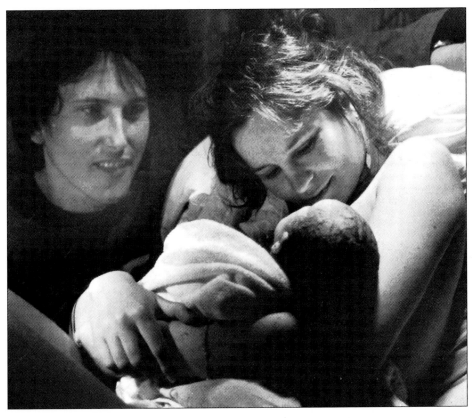

IMPORTANCE OF BONDING

If it seems that I'm emphasizing this bonding process between parent and infant, I feel it's for good reason. Research has shown that parents who are given unrestricted contact with their children immediately after delivery rear their children in a more constructive way, are more sympathetic to problems, ask more questions, give reasons for their actions, and explain situations better than do parents whose babies are taken away at birth. A further part of this research showed that at the age of five years the children who had had extended contact with their parents scored higher in intelligence tests than the control group. This does not mean that good bonding with your infant makes your baby a more intelligent child. What I think it points to is that it makes you a different kind of parent and possibly a better one.

FATHER'S FIRST CONTACT

Paternal bonding with an infant is not very different and certainly just as important as maternal bonding. So during this sensitive period after the birth it's important for you to hold your baby and make eye and skin contact. If you have been present at the birth and comforted your partner throughout the labor, this is a good beginning. Stay with your partner and your baby as long as possible after the birth. Be responsive to the cues that your infant will give you. It may take you a little longer and you may have to fit yourself into the role to achieve the same degree of responsiveness as the mother. All this can be helped by early and extended contact with your baby in her first weeks of life. Very often birth helps a man to express and enjoy emotions that society primes him to repress.

Establishing a routine

THE FIRST FEW DAYS will be hard; labor and birth are physically and emotionally draining. If you are in the hospital you are subject to a certain amount of routine—regular checks by midwives, ward rounds by obstetricians or pediatricians, meals at certain times, visits by physiotherapists, family and friends, and so on—plus learning to feed, change and bathe your baby. I had my first baby in a hospital and expected to have a restful time; instead I hardly had a minute to myself, few minutes alone with my baby and was utterly exhausted at night—I couldn't wait to get home to peace and security.

Even if you have your baby at home, you'll find that one activity succeeds another almost without respite, and all the time you are learning. You may have read all the baby books that are available, but no book tells you about your baby. There's no short cut to learning about your baby's care because you have to take your lead

from her. Babies don't know night from day and they require the same attention during the night as they do during the day.

The smaller your baby, the more often you will have to feed her. Small babies, say 7 lb (3.1 kg) or under, require food at least every four hours and often there may be only three hours or two and a half hours between feeds. You should feed on demand; if you do, your baby will find her own routine faster than if you try to impose your routine on her. At least twice during the night your newborn baby will need a feed and a diaper change. Nearly everyone I have spoken to seems to have had a well-behaved baby who slept for six hours during the night within a week of being delivered. Well, mine didn't! The baby that gives you more than four hours' sleep during the night is an exception.

The best way to manage all that's demanded of you and to stay cheerful and to get enough rest is to take your cue from

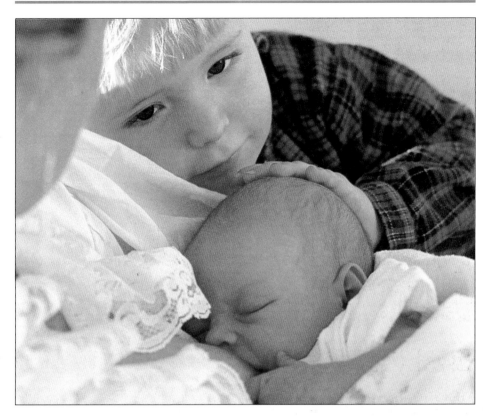

the baby. You're going to have to learn to catnap because the only opportunity you may get to sleep during the first few days is when your baby is asleep. Just after delivery you have little stamina and will easily become exhausted from physical effort. Emotionally you are in a labile state because of the sudden withdrawal of pregnancy hormones. Little problems seem insurmountable and big ones insoluble. You may find yourself short-tempered and irritable with flashes of elation in between. You may be tearful and collapse in a heap as soon as anything goes wrong and the next minute find yourself imbued with strong resolutions. Don't expect too much of yourself.

If you have a home confinement, or an early discharge from the hospital, be easy on yourself. Don't worry about day-to-day domestic chores. Let them pile up; any

NEW MEMBER OF THE FAMILY
When you introduce your new baby to an older child, let him feel and touch her.

outside helper can see to those things. Save your energy to concentrate on what matters, and there really are only a few things that should get top priority: the baby, then you, then your partner and any other children, then all of you as a family unit. Be unscrupulous in asking for help, even if it's only for the first week, so that you have time on your own to get to know your baby and to work your day around her needs.

Most newborn babies have the same basic needs in the first few weeks of life, and once you have established a routine, you can then set about deciding what your needs are and how best to organize yourself on a typical day.

NEWBORN REFLEXES

Babies are born with certain reflexes which help them to survive the first days outside the womb. For example, babies put to the breast immediately after delivery will root for the nipple and suck to get at their mother's milk.

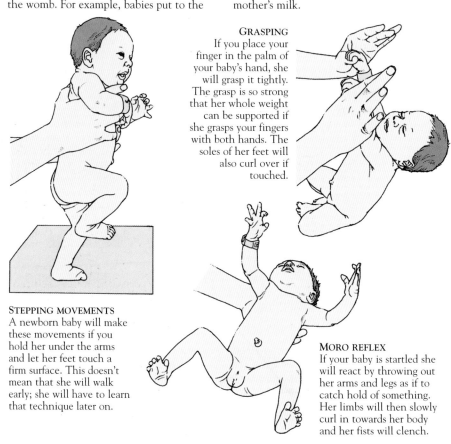

GRASPING
If you place your finger in the palm of your baby's hand, she will grasp it tightly. The grasp is so strong that her whole weight can be supported if she grasps your fingers with both hands. The soles of her feet will also curl over if touched.

STEPPING MOVEMENTS
A newborn baby will make these movements if you hold her under the arms and let her feet touch a firm surface. This doesn't mean that she will walk early; she will have to learn that technique later on.

MORO REFLEX
If your baby is startled she will react by throwing out her arms and legs as if to catch hold of something. Her limbs will then slowly curl in towards her body and her fists will clench.

THE APGAR SCALE

When your baby is born, her condition is assessed according to a series of five standard tests called the Apgar score at one minute and five minutes after the birth. Each test is given a score of 2, 1 or 0. The tests cover:
● heart rate (above 100 beats per minute 2; below 1; absent 0)
● breathing (regular 2; irregular 1; absent 0)
● movements (active 2; some 1; limp 0)
● skin color (pink 2; bluish extremities 1; blue 0)
● reflex response (cries 2; whimpers 1; absent 0).

A score of 7 or over is normal, and a low first score improving to a normal second score is still fine. A low score at the second testing may mean your baby needs the immediate attention of a pediatrician.

The mother

FOR THE FIRST SEVEN DAYS after the birth, whether you are at home or in the hospital, you should stay in bed for as much of the day as possible and sleep and rest whenever the baby sleeps. You will certainly be disappointed at your new shape. Your stomach will have sagged, your breasts will look large now that your bulge has gone and your thighs will seem heavy. Start on your postnatal exercises (see p. 228) right away.

AFTERPAINS

Throughout our fertile lives the uterus never stops contracting; these contractions are felt as menstrual cramps at the time of our periods, as Braxton Hicks contractions throughout pregnancy, and after delivery as afterpains. Uterine contractions after delivery are stronger and more painful than usual because they are the means by which the uterus contracts down to its former nonpregnant size. The faster and harder it contracts down the less likelihood there is of any postpartum hemorrhage (see p. 210). The contractions are usually not severe with the first baby but subsequently women become more conscious of them. They are more severe in breastfeeding women but are an excellent sign that you are getting back to normal quickly. They usually disappear after three or four days.

LOCHIA

For anything up to six weeks you may pass lochia, which is a discharge of blood and mucus from the uterus. Immediately after delivery it is like a pink or red menstrual flow and after a few days it becomes a dark brown and gradually fades to a creamy color and finally becomes white. You should use sanitary pads as protection (superabsorbent ones for the first two days) and delay the use of tampons until after the first full period. Both the

contracting down of the uterus and the cessation of bleeding occur more rapidly if you breastfeed the baby.

BOWELS AND BLADDER

You should use the toilet as soon as you possibly can after delivery. Quite often the bowels have been well cleared out at some point before or during labor and you may not want to pass a bowel motion for 24 hours or more. Don't worry about this but obey the first call to move your bowels and take care not to strain. Drinking water and walking about will help to get your bowels working. There may be some hesitancy before the urine starts to flow. This is nothing to worry about and is usually the result of swelling of the perineum and the tissues that surround the bladder and the urethral opening. A good way to get started is to sit in some warm water, try out the Kegel exercises (see p. 125) and pass urine into the water. This is not unhygienic if you wash yourself thoroughly afterwards. If you've had stitches, passing urine may sting. Try pouring warm water over yourself as you are passing urine to reduce stinging.

You may also notice an increase in the amount of urine passed for the first few days. This is the way your body eliminates the excess fluid you have accumulated during your pregnancy.

COPING WITH STITCHES

Most stitches dissolve after five or six days. If you are bruised or the stitches cause you discomfort:
- sit on an inflatable rubber ring
- after bathing, dry the area thoroughly with a hair dryer
- put salt in the bath to aid healing
- hold a clean pad against the stitches when you move your bowels
- don't get constipated (see p. 148).

Feeding

WHICHEVER METHOD OF feeding you choose, remember the colostrum in your breasts during the first three days contains valuable antibodies that will protect your baby against all kinds of diseases.

BREASTFEEDING

This is something that you have to learn for yourself—no one can give you any lessons. If you are in the hospital, ask the nursing staff to help you to get started.

Establishing breastfeeding is always easier if you put the baby to the breast within a few minutes of delivery (see p. 215). Once you've achieved successful suckling in the happy relaxed atmosphere that surrounds the birth, you'll feel confident about future feeding. If this isn't possible, start feeding as soon as you can and try to relax

SUCCESSFUL BREASTFEEDING
Breastfeeding will go more smoothly if you put your baby to the breast as soon as possible after delivery.

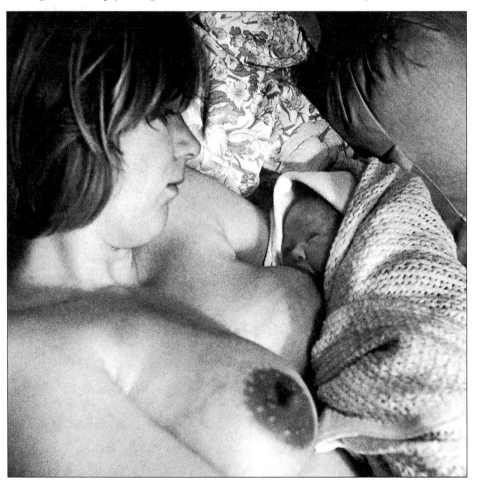

and enjoy the experience. You may feel sore around the nipples, or your baby may not be very good at feeding at first, but it will come in time. Remember every woman is equipped to feed her baby, and no breast is too small to feed a baby. Supply automatically meets demand.

COLOSTRUM

During the first three days the breasts produce light, yellow-colored colostrum. It is a perfect food for the first days of your baby's life. It contains water, protein and minerals in just the right proportion to take care of all your baby's nutritional needs. Colostrum also contains valuable antibodies which protect your baby against diseases to which you have developed a resistance, such as polio and influenza. Besides all that, it contains a laxative that gets your newborn baby's bowels in motion. After about 72 hours, colostrum is replaced by breast milk, and for about two to three days, your breasts will feel heavy and full.

LETDOWN REFLEX

The letdown reflex is the automatic reaction by which the body makes milk available in the breasts. The reflex is a complicated chemical chain reaction that occurs in seconds and is set off either upon stimulation of your nipple by the baby, or by your baby's hunger cry or even by the thought of your baby. At this trigger the pituitary gland releases a hormone, oxytocin, which causes the milk-producing cells to empty their milk into the reservoirs in the nipple area. If you are not ready to feed, press the sides of your breasts firmly to control the flow.

GETTING BREASTFEEDING GOING

In the first days the nipples are delicate and they need time to toughen up so increase the length of time on each breast gradually. Two minutes on each breast will give your baby sufficient colostrum at first. Make sure she is properly latched on (see below). Build up the time on each breast to 10 minutes each side by the time the milk has come in on about the third or fourth day. All babies suck most strongly in the first five minutes, during which they take about 80 percent of the feed. When she has had enough, she'll lose interest and start to play with your breast. She may turn away and fall asleep. You'll know if she hasn't had enough because she will awake hungry and cry. At the next feed, alternate the breast you start on.

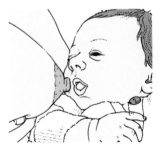

ROOTING REFLEX
If you touch the baby's cheek with your nipple or finger, she will turn towards the breast and try to latch on. This is known as the rooting reflex. It is instinctive and can be further encouraged if you express colostrum onto the baby's lips.

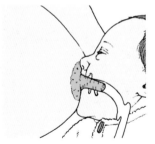

LATCHING ON
The baby is properly latched on when she has the whole of the nipple area in her mouth, with her tongue underneath the nipple. She presses the top of her mouth against the milk reservoirs (see p. 95).

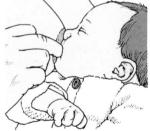

BREAKING THE SUCTION
At the end of a feed don't pull your breast away from the baby. This will make your nipple sore. Instead insert your finger into the corner of her mouth and gently ease her off the breast, or press down on her chin.

BREAST CARE

You will need to take care of your breasts during the early days. Buy at least two of the best maternity bras that you can afford (see p. 137) and pay strict attention to the daily hygiene of your breasts and nipples. Bathe them every day with water; don't use soap because it defats the skin and can encourage a crack or a sore to develop. Always handle your breasts with care. Never rub them dry, always pat dry.

After feeding, if possible, leave your nipples open to the air for a short time. Wear pads inside your bra to soak up any milk that may leak, and change these pads often. Don't leave a wet pad in contact with your breast for any length of time. To avoid cracked nipples, apply a drop of oil or cream (arachis oil or olive oil or hypericum calendula cream) to the pad.

TIPS ON BREASTFEEDING

- Give yourself time to prepare for feeding. Have a comfortable chair ready, and surround yourself with everything you need. If you're in bed, prop yourself up with pillows.
- Hold the baby high enough so that she can reach the nipple without effort. Cradle her head in the crook of your arm, and support her back and bottom with your lower arm and hand.
- Relax your shoulders. If you have to bend your back to lower the nipple to the baby, you will quickly become tired and your neck and shoulders will tense up.
- If your breasts become full of milk soon after a feed, express a little (see p. 236) to help you to feel more comfortable.
- If your breasts are full and hard, the nipple will flatten out and the baby will have difficulty latching on. Express a little milk to soften the areola and as the milk flows the baby will latch on and suck.
- If you get too tired, you can express some milk and put it in a bottle for your partner or a friend to give to the baby.
- To ease engorgement, apply hot or cold cloths to your breasts and with gentle massage the milk will flow.
- If you develop a crack, express from the sore breast until the skin heals. Give the baby the expressed milk from a spoon if you don't want to bother with bottles and sterilization.
- If the baby refuses the breast it may be because she is having difficulty in breathing. Press down on the top of your breast gently with a finger to clear a space for her nostrils.
- If you feel feverish and notice a shiny, red patch on your breast, consult your doctor. This could be a blocked duct.

BURPING

Some babies swallow enough air during feeding to cause them discomfort, and their piercing screams after a feed are silenced as soon as the wind is passed. Other babies are never bothered by wind. If you aren't sure, hold your baby in a upright position and pat her back. If nothing happens, and the baby is happy, there is no need to wait for a burp. Your baby may regurgitate (spit-up) a little milk when she burps. Some babies spit-up, others don't. The commonest cause is overfeeding, and there is nothing to worry about even if it looks a lot. Have a cotton diaper ready or put a bib on the baby.

BOTTLE FEEDING

If you have decided to bottle feed your baby, you will experience about two uncomfortable days while the milk dries up in your breasts. You will be advised to wear a good, firm bra and to take mild analgesics if necessary to relieve the pain of engorgement. By the fifth day after your baby's birth, your breasts should be back to normal.

The main advantage of bottle feeding is that the new father can be involved right from the beginning with feeding and feeding-time activities. When either of you feeds your baby, make sure your back is supported and hold the bottle firmly at an angle so that the teat is always full of milk. If not, the baby will suck in air with her feed. The teat should be well back in the baby's mouth. If your baby shows no interest in feeding, encourage her to "root" (see p. 221) for the bottle by gently touching her cheek with your finger or the teat. If the teat suddenly goes flat, release the vacuum by gently pulling on the bottle, to allow the milk to flow again. Sometimes the teat becomes blocked; change it for a new, sterile one.

MAKING EYE CONTACT
Always try to hold your baby while you feed her so that she can see your face.

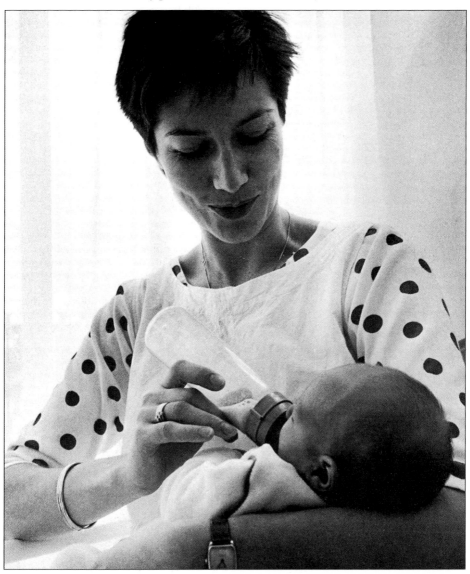

Bathing and changing

UNTIL YOUR BABY IS six weeks old, the only parts that need daily bathing are the head, hands and bottom. To do this you need to "top and tail." Try to make it approximately the same time every day so that you can both establish a routine.

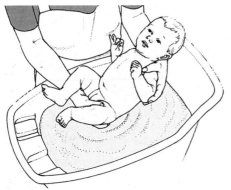

IN THE BATH
Support your baby's head with your forearm and her bottom with your other hand. Her head should be slightly upright, enabling her to look around. You can even start playing water games.

TIPS FOR BATHTIME

● Warm the room to at least 68°F (20°C) and use water that is about 90°F (32°C) so that it is warm and not hot when you dip your elbow into it.
● Squeeze just a drop of liquid baby soap into the bath if you want suds. Even the mildest soap is defatting and dries the skin.
● Try to bathe your baby at a time when you will not be disturbed. Make sure all the baby's things are ready and at hand before you start, otherwise you won't be able to reach them because your hands will be full with the baby.
● Wear a waterproof apron with a towel tied around your waist so that you can slip the wet baby straight onto your knee.

TOPPING AND TAILING

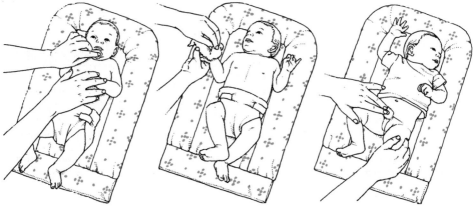

1 Fill a bowl with warm boiled water and place cotton wool beside it. Undress the baby, except for her diaper, and wipe each eye with a separate piece of cotton wool dipped in the water and squeezed dry. Wipe from the inside of the eye outwards.

2 Take another piece of cotton wool and use it to wipe around the creases of her neck, behind her ears, her face, and mouth and nostrils. Don't clean inside her ears. Pat the skin dry with a soft towel and wipe her hands and arms with a facecloth.

3 Put on a clean undershirt and remove her diaper. With a new piece of cotton wool, wipe all around the genital area, especially between the creases. Dry her skin thoroughly. Most babies enjoy the freedom of not having a diaper on for a time.

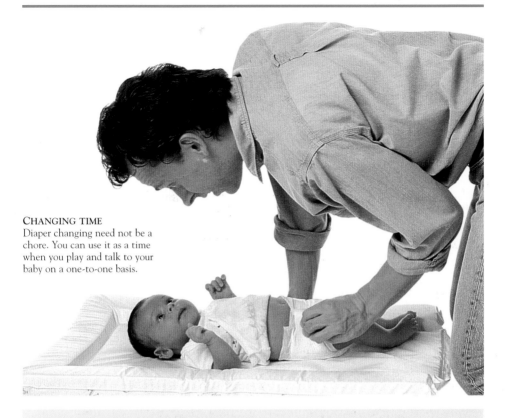

CHANGING TIME
Diaper changing need not be a chore. You can use it as a time when you play and talk to your baby on a one-to-one basis.

REUSABLE OR DISPOSABLE DIAPERS?

There are many issues that you will have to think about when you are deciding whether to opt for disposable or reusable diapers.

Many parents have given up using fabric diapers, not only because disposables are so much more convenient but also because traditional cotton squares can be uncomfortable, particularly for newborn babies, who have such delicate skin. Cloth diapers can also be time-consuming to put on, particularly for parents of a newborn baby, who may be changing their baby's diaper at every feed and sometimes in between. New parents are also sometimes nervous of dealing with diaper pins.

When deciding whether to use disposable or reusable diapers, it's important to weigh up the costs. After all, your baby will be using diapers for at least two years. As well

as the cost of the diapers themselves, there are other costs associated with reusable diapers, including the cost of washing powder, electricity, sanitizing fluid and items such as diaper buckets. However, the cost of disposables can mount up, and modern reusable diapers are much less bulky than the old-fashioned type. They are usually shaped, and many types have built-in strong Velcro fasteners, or you can use pinless fasteners so that you don't have to worry about using safety pins.

If you decide to opt for reusable diapers, it's a good idea also to use disposable or reusable liners to avoid heavy soiling with feces. Reusable diapers should be soaked for several hours in a covered bucket in sanitizing fluid before being boiled or machine-washed at the hottest setting.

Postpartum blues

WEEPINESS AND DEPRESSION are common around the third or fourth day when the milk starts to flow. If you find that your depression is more than just feeling a bit low and it lasts longer than two weeks, you should seek medical help immediately. Don't allow the depression to drag on thinking that it will disappear. Early medical help may defuse the situation, and going without help may make your depression worse and mean that it will take longer for you to feel better.

Like any other depression, postpartum depression is more likely the wider the disparity between expectations and reality. Any negative feelings you may have, whether it is about yourself or the baby or about motherhood, will be exaggerated in the early days because of the fragile emotional state you are in. It's the fault of your hormones which, after having been at very high levels for nine months, are suddenly plunged back to the comparatively low levels of normality. This enormous swing renders most women tearful, weepy, irritable, indecisive, moody, uncommunicative, anxious, insomniac and depressed. After the initial euphoria has worn off, reality seems difficult to cope with. You'd be absolutely wrong to think that the early days are easy. They are not. You'd be wrong to think that you have a lead on every woman and know how to manage the early days. No one does. The expertise, the tricks, the responsibilities of motherhood are acquired only through learning, which takes time, so be easy on yourself. Gather as much information as you can, talk to the midwife, the doctor, to friends who have had babies and to experienced mothers. Relieve yourself of unimportant tasks.

Don't try to keep up appearances. Let everybody but the baby and your partner fend for themselves. Be as open as your personality allows you to be. Consult your partner and friends about worries and problems. One of the best ways to keep the stresses, strains and new responsibilities of motherhood in perspective and prevent them escalating into a serious emotional disturbance is to talk.

REST AND SLEEP

Sufficient rest and sleep in the first few days are essential though difficult to achieve. Many women feel exhausted after childbirth; it seems that your body is letting you down because it simply cannot function the way it did before you were pregnant. One of the reasons why you feel so exhausted is that the volume of your blood has been suddenly cut by 30 percent. Therefore a sufficient volume of blood cannot reach your muscles for them to work efficiently and so they feel weak and tire easily. It will take you several weeks to readjust to this enormous change. I well remember going shopping five days after delivery to get a few things for the baby. I didn't have to walk far to the shops and I wasn't carrying anything heavy but before I got back to my car, I had to sit down and rest. This is normal and you should try to avoid even moderate activity.

GETTING ENOUGH REST

● Never ignore signs of tiredness. Stop whatever you are doing, if it isn't essential, and lie down with your feet raised slightly above your head.
● You don't have to go to sleep to conserve your strength; resting will give your heart, lungs and other vital organs time to recover.
● Whether you have had a hospital or a home birth, have someone to help with the household chores and the baby so that you can rest during the day.
● Discourage visitors if you feel unable to cope. Put yourself and the baby first and ask to be left alone.

MOTHER-LOVE

Everyone thinks that mother-love comes readymade with breast milk. This is not so. Many women would admit that they feel very little in terms of deep love for their baby within the first 24–48 hours. Love has to grow and the bonding process takes time. There is nothing wrong with you if it takes several days or even a couple of weeks. Mother-love is not something that can be pre-arranged, and feelings of caring, protectiveness and love for your new baby have to develop in their own time.

COPING WITH BEING IN HOSPITAL

It may appear that the maternity ward is being run for the convenience of nurses and doctors rather than for mothers and babies and to a degree this is true. You may not take easily to quite a lot that happens in a hospital. Midwives may be busy and possibly overworked, and may not be able to give you as much time or help as you need. A hospital diet is not exciting and you may find the food badly cooked or too bland for your taste. Visitors can tire you out as well, so most maternity units now restrict visiting (except for fathers); your partner needs to be alert

and tactfully to suggest that friends and family stagger their visits to start off with. On the other hand there is quite a lot to enjoy while you are in a hospital. You'll have company and can share your experiences, observations and worries with other mothers. A pleasant social life can develop between mothers with new babies and you may form new friendships which will last well after confinement. There is a lot to be said for the companionship and friendliness that exist between mothers in maternity wards.

If ward life doesn't suit you, you can make your feelings known to the nursing staff. There are many ward sisters who take an enlightened and flexible view and will do their best to accommodate you. If this isn't possible, you will find that your unhappiness deepens. It would be sad if the first few days with your baby were marred by the frustrations of hospital life, so it would probably be better for all concerned if you asked for a discharge from the hospital and, if necessary, took your own discharge. If you feel that you haven't the strength of mind to make a decision like this, consult your partner and ask him to make a firm decision. The probability is that he will advise you to come home. In this case, don't prevaricate, do as he says.

LEAVING THE HOSPITAL

Hospital practice varies, but whether you leave the hospital after 24 hours or five days, some of the following procedures will apply to your discharge.

- A doctor will give you a physical examination to check your breasts and to see that your uterus is returning to its pre-pregnant size and that your stitches are healing. The lochia will also be inspected to see if you have passed any blood clots.
- You will be asked about contraception, and you will be given a prescription if you need one. If you are breastfeeding, a low dose pill will be prescribed (see p. 235).
- If you weren't immune to rubella

(see p. 36) during your pregnancy, ask to be immunized before you leave hospital. The vaccination will not affect the baby if you are breastfeeding.
- The midwife will show you how to clean the baby's umbilical cord if it has not already dropped off.
- The baby will be checked by a pediatrician; if you have any worries, ask now. You will be advised to take your baby to a clinic for a six-week developmental check-up.
- You will be given a date for your postnatal checkup or advised to see your doctor near to that date.

POSTNATAL EXERCISES

Exercise at least once a day as soon as you can after delivery. It is, however, better to exercise for a short time, say five minutes, several times a day. Lie on your stomach for the first few days too, to help bring the uterus forward into its prepregnant position.

THE FIRST DAYS

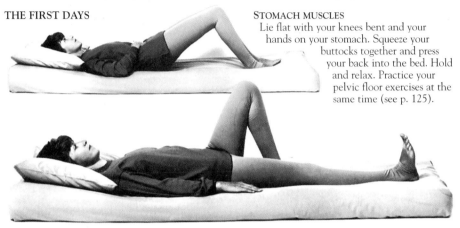

STOMACH MUSCLES

Lie flat with your knees bent and your hands on your stomach. Squeeze your buttocks together and press your back into the bed. Hold and relax. Practice your pelvic floor exercises at the same time (see p. 125).

HIP HITCHING

Lie on your back, bend one knee and flex the foot of the straight leg. Lengthen that straight leg by pushing your heel away from you. Then shorten it by bringing it up towards you (without bending your knee). Make sure you don't arch your back.

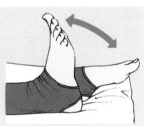

FOOT PEDALING

Flex your foot up and down as if you were pedaling. This is one of the first exercises you can do after delivery. It encourages good circulation and prevents your ankles and feet from swelling.

BASIC ROUTINE

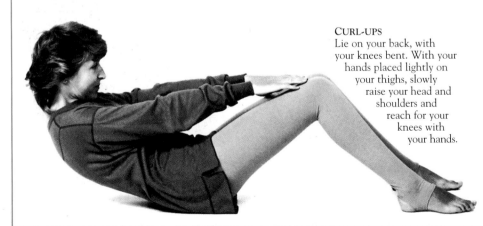

CURL-UPS

Lie on your back, with your knees bent. With your hands placed lightly on your thighs, slowly raise your head and shoulders and reach for your knees with your hands.

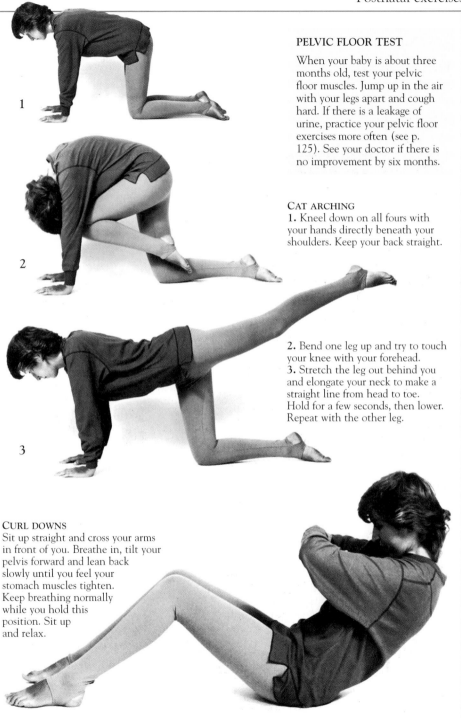

PELVIC FLOOR TEST

When your baby is about three months old, test your pelvic floor muscles. Jump up in the air with your legs apart and cough hard. If there is a leakage of urine, practice your pelvic floor exercises more often (see p. 125). See your doctor if there is no improvement by six months.

CAT ARCHING

1. Kneel down on all fours with your hands directly beneath your shoulders. Keep your back straight.

2. Bend one leg up and try to touch your knee with your forehead.
3. Stretch the leg out behind you and elongate your neck to make a straight line from head to toe. Hold for a few seconds, then lower. Repeat with the other leg.

CURL DOWNS

Sit up straight and cross your arms in front of you. Breathe in, tilt your pelvis forward and lean back slowly until you feel your stomach muscles tighten. Keep breathing normally while you hold this position. Sit up and relax.

18

Getting back to normal

Every woman feels differently after the birth of her baby. If the weather is warm and sunny, you may feel like getting up and sitting outside with the baby in the carriage beside you; if it is cold and wintry outside, the coziness of your room will be what you seek. However, you should give yourself at least 7–10 days to build up enough strength before you get back to the normal routines.

Coming home from the hospital is exciting; you'll feel comforted and confident to be back amongst familiar surroundings, though it can be somewhat disorientating. As time goes on, if you don't make plans to meet people, you may feel isolated. However, the birth of your baby could open many doors to you. You'll find that getting out and about with your baby can create a new way of life within your local community.

The new family

HOW MUCH YOU AND YOUR baby will have established a routine depends largely on how long you stayed in a hospital. A stay of three to five days allows you to get to know each other and, taking the lead from your baby, you will have probably formed a loose timetable to suit his needs (see p. 216). On the other hand, if you leave a hospital within the first day or two after delivery or if you had a home birth, your routines will be initiated at home and will be based on the day-to-day running of the household. There has to be give and take on both sides; the baby is an important member of the household, but

he also has to fit in with other members of the family and their needs. There's no question in my mind that the quickest way to establish a routine is to let your baby lead you and to organize yourself, your life and your interests into the time that he leaves you free to do so, after you have taken care of all his needs. It's easiest on the whole household if you wait and see how often the baby wants to feed, how often he wants to sleep, when his usual waking times and sleeping times are, and try to dovetail your chores around his clock. One of the most important things for you to note is your baby's longest sleeping time. Try to fit in a nap or a rest during the same time. Establishing a routine does not mean "training" your baby to eat, sleep and play according to a timetable that suits you. What it really means is feeding and playing with your baby when he's awake, trying to rest when he's asleep and fitting the rest of your life around his daily routine.

One of the early ways to introduce the baby to a diurnal rhythm is to make night feeds quiet and in a low light with as little disruption as possible. The daylight hours will then become synonymous in his mind with bustle and noise.

MEETING OTHER CHILDREN

If you have another child (or children) and are not having your baby at home, it is worth thinking carefully about how you are going to introduce your child to a new baby and so help to avoid jealousy. When you first greet him, make sure that someone else is carrying the baby so that your arms are free to hold out, welcome him and gather him up for a cuddle. For the first few minutes give him all your attention, just as you would if you had been apart for any other reason.

Bring a present from the newborn baby—something that your child has really been looking forward to having. If he is physically capable, let him hold the newborn baby himself. Most young children are anxious to be of help, so encourage your child to give you all the assistance he can. During the first days and weeks, set aside some times, several during the day if you can, which are just for you and him to be together, and which even the baby can't interrupt.

Don't break old habits just because the baby has come. So, if you had a special routine at breakfast time or bedtime, continue it with your child if you possibly can. Feed the baby just before these special times, so you won't be interrupted. When you have visitors, don't let them pay all their attention to the newborn

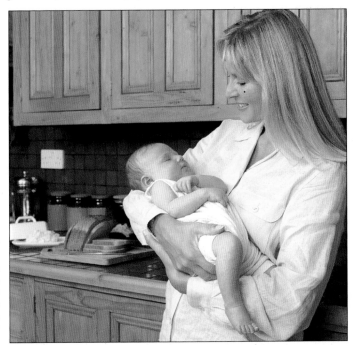

LIFE WITH YOUR BABY
As you become more confident, you'll find that it becomes natural to integrate your baby into your daily routine at home, and you'll start to enjoy his company more and more.

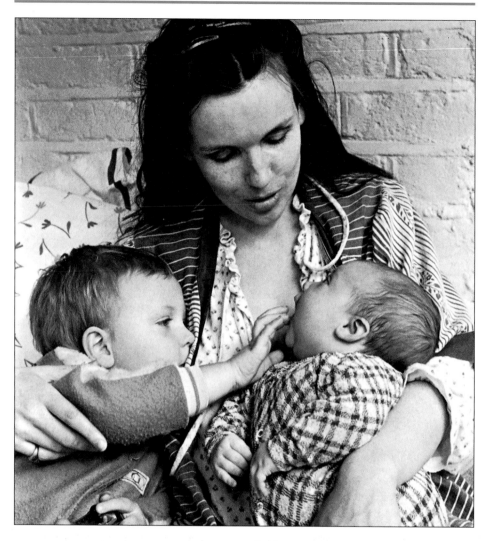

INTEGRATING YOUR FAMILY
Closeness and involvement will help your toddler to accept the new baby without feeling shut out of your world.

baby; try to make sure that your child has at least as much. It also helps if you can praise and reward him as much as you possibly can and keep scolding to a minimum in the first few weeks. If you are going to be in a hospital for several days, try to make arrangements so that your child can come into the hospital to see you and the baby as soon as possible after delivery and regularly thereafter.

RELATIONSHIP WITH YOUR PARTNER

With a new baby, a mother starts out on an exciting relationship with another person and may feel little sense of loss when the closeness with her partner gradually diminishes. This is not so for a father and a woman should remember

TIPS FOR COPING WITH TIREDNESS

Even if your baby sleeps well between feeds, your body needs to recover from the birth, and you will suffer from fatigue, particularly in the afternoon. To keep up your strength and good spirits and to get back to normal quickly, get as much rest as you can.

● Have a rest whenever the baby is sleeping; don't use this time for chores.

● If you aren't feeling well, don't be stoical, call your doctor. Your health could get worse.

● Continue to take any prescribed iron pills for at least six weeks.

● Keep to the balanced diet you had during pregnancy (see pp. 108–116) and pay particular attention to what you eat if you are breastfeeding. This is not a good time to diet. Breastfeeding in itself uses up fat laid down for the purpose during pregnancy.

● Drink lots of fluids; you will feel very thirsty if you are breastfeeding.

● Have meals and snacks that require the minimum of preparation such as salads, cheese, wholegrain-bread sandwiches, fresh fruit and yogurt.

● Take all the short cuts you can think of.

● Use only disposable diapers at first.

● Accept any offers of help for cooking and cleaning, so that you can relax and enjoy the baby.

● Let your older children help with the baby—tidying the crib or folding away diapers.

● Keep the baby in the room with you for the first few weeks. You won't have to go far to pick him up and you can keep him in bed with you if you want to.

● Keep a couple of diapers in the kitchen, the car, the bathroom and the baby's room so you don't have to go back to the nursery at every diaper change.

● Believe in the fact that you need help.

this. A man's jealousy of his baby is not uncommon and many men confess to feeling pushed out by the baby and neglected by their partners. You must make sure that both of you understand that it is inevitable in the early days for the baby to become the main focus of attention. Therefore you should both make time for each other. One way to resume your closeness is to take a nap together at the end of the working day.

One of the adjustments you both have to make is that no part of your life can be as spontaneous as it was before the baby. You both need to become more flexible and possibly more tolerant than you were before, being ready to give time and attention to each other when the opportunity arises. Look for the opportunities or you may find that all your attention is going to the baby without you even realizing it.

You'll also realize that you begin to feel differently about each other. This doesn't mean less, just different. It isn't a sign that your relationship is deteriorating; it is more likely to mature and become richer.

Don't keep wishing that it was the same as before, because it never can be.

ADJUSTMENT TO FATHERHOOD

If you're relaxed and confident about the newborn baby, you will enjoy family life much more and your involvement will help you to appreciate that looking after a baby is every bit as exhausting as a day at the office or factory.

● Bathe and change the baby within the first few days and keep it up to give yourself confidence.

● Spend as much time as you can with your baby. Assert your right to have the baby to yourself for a time—your partner will be glad of the break.

● Talk to your employers about the new addition to your family. If you have to get away early or adopt more flexible working hours in the first few months, they may be more amenable if they have had prior warning of your changed circumstances and you will know where you stand in relation to paternity leave.

Resuming sexual relations

YOUR RELATIONSHIP with your partner changes in all sorts of ways and for most people this includes sex. In the first few months after the birth, sex can become a bit of a problem and can make you feel depressed about your new role. Some women lose their sex drive for a couple of months after childbirth and sometimes for longer. It's not uncommon for fathers to feel the same and to lose their ability to maintain an erection. Both of you must be prepared for this change of feeling and not to take it personally. If you both can be philosophical and loving about your problems, you'll prevent them developing into long-term obstacles.

WHEN TO RESUME SEX

There is no magic date when you can start to have sexual relations again. It will help if you start your pelvic floor exercises (see p. 125) immediately after delivery, even though your genital area may be a bit sore. Take it slowly and gently. The ideal time to start making love again is when you and your partner want to, so discuss it and try it out tentatively. You may find that the tissues are a bit sore or tight but waiting will not make them stretch. Glands that normally lubricate the vaginal area sometimes don't function for a short while after delivery, so use a lubricating cream or jelly. It helps, too, if the vagina is well relaxed before penetration, so concentrate on foreplay before sexual intercourse. Try a different position from the woman lying on her back as the penis can press on the rear wall of the vagina, which may still be sensitive and slightly bruised. Your partner can help by gentle manual dilatation if your vagina seems to be too tight. Don't be concerned about setbacks—they're normal; try again gently.

Many couples resume sex at the time of the postnatal checkup. If you've had an episiotomy you'll be sore and tender for

longer and your partner should not attempt penetration until you feel comfortable. However, this does not disbar gentle exploration. Also, while you are breast-feeding, your breasts may feel sore and heavy, and if you have a cracked nipple, fondling will be out of the question.

If after several months one of you is still feeling reluctant to resume your sexual relationship, do ask for help. You'll be surprised how much easier it is once you've talked to someone, and it may be easier for you both to talk with a third party, perhaps a friend or a relative or a sex counselor. The most important thing is to talk about your feelings.

LOSS OF LIBIDO

● Many women feel unattractive for a while after childbirth; your body will still be a bit shapeless compared to your pre-pregnancy figure. It's difficult to feel sexually attractive if you have a poor self-image (see p. 102).

● The presence of the baby may be a stumbling block to expressions of love and sexual interest, especially if he is sleeping in the same room.

● You will both be feeling tired and fatigue does tend to inhibit normal sexual urges. Try to get as much rest as possible.

● Particularly if you had an episiotomy or a cesarean, your scar will take a while to heal and you may be loath to try having sex for the time being.

● Parents do become very baby-orientated in the first few weeks, and you may feel that there isn't room for anyone else in your emotions. This is perfectly natural. What you should do is tell your partner about your feelings. You'll probably both feel this way to some degree.

● Many of the daily activities surrounding babies may make you feel unattractive—washing diapers, and smells of spit-up—all these things can be a bit off-putting.

CONTRACEPTION

Even if you are breastfeeding, or haven't restarted menstruating, you are unprotected and should use some form of contraception when you resume intercourse. If you breastfeed your baby totally, your periods will probably not return until you wean him; if you don't breastfeed, or only for a short time, your periods should return between two and four months. You will be asked before you are discharged from the hospital about your planned form of contraception and you may want to organize it at this time rather than wait until your postnatal checkup, which is usually between four and six weeks after the birth.

The pill

The pill is not usually prescribed until three weeks after your birth. If you are breastfeeding, you will be prescribed a progesterone-only "mini-pill." This contains no estrogen, which interferes with your metabolism and could have an inhibiting effect on milk production. The mini-pill is not 100 percent reliable, however; you must take one pill every day at around the same time to be sure. The hormones in the mini-pill are also secreted in your milk, and it is not yet known if this has any effects on the baby. However, this method is recommended while breastfeeding. During your pregnancy and after the birth you may have suffered certain conditions for the first time. You would be unwise to use the contraceptive pill if you have high blood pressure, diabetes or postnatal depression.

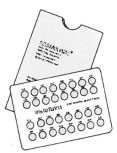

CONTRACEPTIVE PILLS

Cap or diaphragm

You will have to be fitted for a new, larger cap as your old one will no longer be reliable. Use it in conjunction with a spermicidal cream or jelly. You will not be fitted for a new cap until your postnatal checkup, about six weeks after the birth. You should have the size checked again around six to nine months in case you need another change in size. If you're happy with it, this method is ideal for the somewhat sporadic lovemaking of new parents.

CAP (DIAPHRAGM)

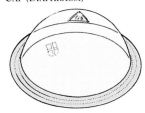

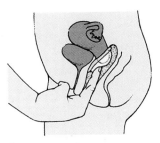

CHECKING POSITION OF CAP
Before you have sexual intercourse always check that the rubber dome of the cap covers the cervix completely.

Intrauterine contraceptive device (IUD)

An IUD can be inserted at your postnatal checkup. The insertion of an IUD is much easier once you've had a baby.

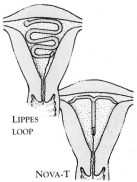

LIPPES
LOOP

NOVA-T

Condom (sheath)

This is the easiest method to use before your checkup. Use plenty of spermicidal jelly or cream with the sheath as your vagina will be less well lubricated.

Injections

There is a contraceptive injection available that is recommended by the manufacturers for women who are forgetful. Having been involved in research into these injections, I know some women may have problems with breakthrough bleeding and a return to fertility after three months is not guaranteed for everyone.

Postnatal checkup

YOUR CHECKUP is usually done about six weeks after delivery at a postnatal clinic at the hospital or at your doctor's office. The purpose of this checkup is to give you a thorough medical and obstetric examination to make sure everything has returned to normal. Your baby is also checked at six weeks, either at a special baby clinic or at your doctor's surgery. If there was any cause for concern at birth you may be asked to bring your baby back to the hospital for his check.

When you go for your checkup, use the opportunity to ask questions about anything that is bothering you, sort out problems and gain reassurance about things that may be causing you anxiety. These questions can be about any subject, about the baby, your own well-being, sex, feeding, crying, routines—about anything that you feel needs clarifying.

During your own medical checkup your blood pressure will be checked and your weight will be noted, your nipples and breasts will be examined, your abdomen will be palpated to check that the uterus has contracted down to its prepregnant size, and you'll have an internal examination and a smear test for cancer of the cervix. If you're suffering from any bladder discomfort or pain when you move your bowels, you should alert your doctor. You should also discuss contraception (see p. 235). A perfect time to have an IUD or a diaphragm fitted is during the internal examination. The doctor will also check the scar if you had any stitching.

THE BABY'S SIX-WEEK CHECK

It is usual for the baby to be weighed and to have his eyes, cord, genitalia and skin checked and for you to have a general discussion with the midwife or doctor about how feeding is going. This would be the time to raise any queries you might have about the daily care of the baby and what you might expect to happen over the next few weeks and months.

Going back to work

HAVING COMMITTED YOURSELF to going back to work while you were pregnant (see p. 52), you may now need to rethink your decision, depending on your emotional and financial circumstances. You should also consult your doctor, who can advise you about factors affecting your health and that of the baby. You should start finding a good system of childcare about six weeks before you intend to return to work, and begin weaning the baby off the breast then, too, at least during the day.

If you begin working before the baby is four months old, and therefore before any mixed feeding, you will need to plan. Try to introduce a routine so that feeding times are predictable and constant. Feed

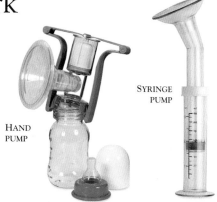

SYRINGE PUMP

HAND PUMP

BREAST PUMPS
If you are working, you may wish to express breast milk so that your childcare provider can feed the baby. You fit the funnel of the pump over the areola and operate the lever or syringe to express the milk.

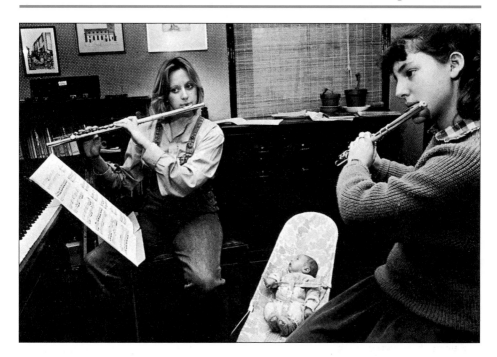

the baby at breakfast and around 6 p.m.; then the person who looks after him need give only the expressed milk or milk substitute for the other two daytime feeds. If you don't want your baby to take any milk substitutes, freeze expressed breast milk; it will keep for up to six months in the freezer. It should take around two weeks to get into this routine. You will need to run down your daytime milk production before returning to work or you will be most uncomfortable during the day.

FINDING GOOD CHILDCARE

You should ask your friends, neighbors, the local council and independent groups what kind of childcare is available in your area. The options may include:
• Childcare providers—women who look after children in their own homes. Ask your Social Services department for a list or take the advice of your pediatrician, and always visit a childcare provider before you put your baby or child into her care.

WORKING FROM HOME
If you are lucky enough to have freelance work in your own home, your baby can stay with you.

• Daycare centers—these are usually run privately. Private daycare centers may be quite expensive, and they may have long waiting lists and usually only a small number of places for babies.
• Nannies— usually young women with a nursery nurses' qualification. They may live in or come to your home on a daily basis. Trained nannies are often the most reliable option for mothers returning to work full time, especially while their babies are still young.
• Au pairs—untrained girls and young women who live with you and help with childcare, babysitting and light housework. They should not be expected to take on the sole care of a young baby for any length of time.
• Workplace daycare—ideal if you want to continue to breastfeed after you return to work. Unfortunately they are still rare.

Enjoying parenthood

I HAVE SPOKEN to many mothers who feel that they have reached the end of their rope within the first few weeks of having a baby. It is important for you to release your pent-up feelings and ease tension and anxiety and enjoy being a parent.

● You really don't have to worry about giving baby care a high priority, you automatically will. You do have to make an effort, though, to give care of yourself a higher priority than most reasonable women want to do. Try to be a little more selfish than you want to be by replacing the less important baby-care activities with care of yourself. Your ultimate aim should be your own peace of mind and happiness. This is particularly important if you are breastfeeding; it is essential that you are fit and rested.

● Even in the early days when you're drawn to be with your baby most of the time, it's essential to have some time on your own, so do whatever you have to do to get it. Perhaps you could arrange with a friend to leave your baby with her for an afternoon a week, and you can do the same for her. You might like to make this a permanent arrangement.

● Don't isolate yourself for too long. Often during the early weeks, you may feel agoraphobic and want to keep safe inside the house with your baby, away from traffic noise and the outside world. If this is your first child, you will soon build up a circle of contacts, either through an independent group or through making friends with other women in the hospital. You could join or set up a babysitting circle in your area.

● Find out about the playgroups and community centers in your area and see what they have to offer. There may be babysitting facilities while you attend a dance class or go shopping.

● Don't expect too much of yourself or of your baby. You aren't perfect, but neither is your baby and you have to forgive imperfections in him as well as yourself. Don't set impossibly high standards of mother or baby behavior. Be prepared to be as flexible as you possibly can.

● Most people find the first early weeks with a baby scary. I did with each of my children and longed for reassurance from the midwife. What you can rest on is the sure knowledge that mothers have taken care of their infants instinctively for millennia, and you are endowed with the same abilities as those mothers.

CRYING

Babies sleep a lot during the first few months, but they also cry a lot as well. Crying is their only means of communication and may be for any number of causes. Check the following:

● Is he hungry? Even if he only fed two hours ago, he might want some more.

● Check his diaper; it could be uncomfortably wet or soiled.

● Is his room warm enough or is he too hot? Babies need a constant temperature of about 65–68°F (18–20°C). If he is too hot, remove some of the covers.

● He may be bored and lonely and want company.

● If your baby mainly cries for prolonged periods at a particular time of day—especially in the evening—it may be what is often known as colic. No one quite knows what causes this typical pattern of crying, during which the baby is difficult to console and may draw his legs up to his chest as though he has a tummy ache. Ask your health visitor to advise you on the best way to soothe him—don't hesitate to use a pacifier if that helps—and hang on to the fact that babies generally grow out of colic by three to four months of age.

YOUR GROWING FAMILY
A contented new family member brings a happy ending to the months of planning and preparation.

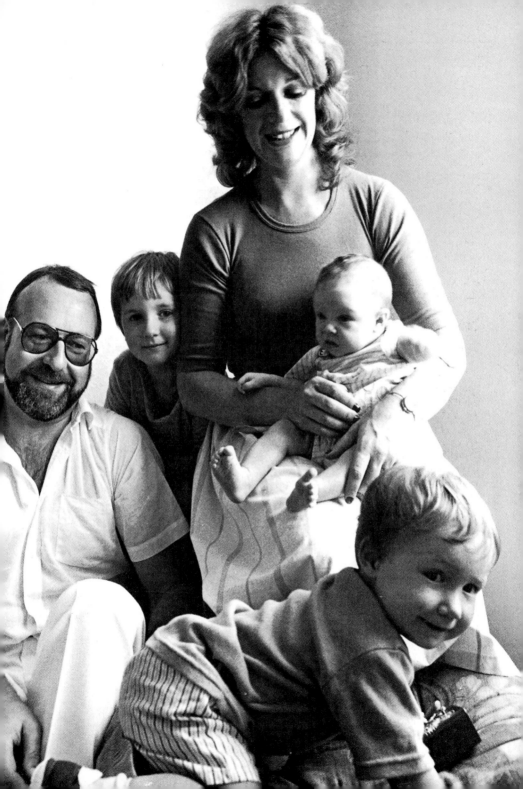

A birthplan

The nine months of your pregnancy will be a time of decision making and preparation. You may already have strong views about how your labor and birth should be managed, or you may be guided by friends who have already had babies and the medical staff who are caring for you. There are a number of choices (see pp. 54–69), and once you have considered the issues and decided what sort of birth you would ideally like, you can write them down in note form on a birthplan.

BIRTHPLAN

Name: Annette Gale
Doctor: Dr. Carrington
Midwife: Sally Lord

Birth attendant

My partner very much wants to be present but he feels some trepidation and would prefer not to be the only birth attendant, so I would like my friend Sally to be there too. She has had three children herself and is a calm person. I would like one of them to be there throughout.

Pain relief

I would like to try to manage without but would not object to trying a TENS machine. I'd like the use of a birthing pool if available. My partner has practiced aromatherapy massage and I would like to try this for the first stage. If I don't feel that I am managing and the labor is going on a long time, please advise me on having an epidural.

Managing labor

I really want to walk around so please don't link me to a belt monitor unless it is medically necessary for the safety of my baby. I would like to arrange to bring in some big cushions to lean on during labor. My two birth attendants can perhaps support me at times.

Position for birth

I really want to squat to deliver. That is why my friend Sally could be so useful as she and my partner could hold me on either side. I haven't tried a birthing stool but if you had one free, I could also try that. If I'm too tired, I would like to deliver on all fours on the floor or on the bed.

Most hospital notes now have a space in which to set down your preferences. Don't worry if you change your mind, as your birth plan can be amended at any prenatal appointment.

There is no guarantee that everything will go exactly as you expect during your labor and birth, and it's helpful to discuss your approach with the midwife at the prenatal clinic, or your doctor, so that they can support you in your decision. If the midwife who attends your labor is not someone you know well from the prenatal clinic, make sure she has seen your birthplan. Here is a sample birthplan for you to consider. Overleaf is a blank plan on which you can write your preferences.

Medical routines

If I have to be induced, I would prefer if it could be done by first trying prostaglandin suppositories, then by rupturing the membranes. If these do not speed things up, I'll take medical advice but I would prefer not to be induced by intravenous drip. I didn't tear last time so I'd prefer not to have an episiotomy unless forceps are needed.

The birth

I regretted not putting my hand down last time to touch the baby's head, so I would like to do that this time. Could you let me know when it appears? Then please put my baby on my tummy afterwards. I do not object to the injected drug that speeds up the third stage.

Breastfeeding

I would like to put the baby to my breast as soon as possible. If the baby has to go to a special unit for any reason, I would want to express milk and get breastfeeding going.

Unforeseen problems

• If I have to have an emergency cesarean, can my husband hold the baby until I come to?
• If the labor is long and I am tiring or the baby is becoming distressed, I will be happy for you to accelerate labor.

Notes

• I would like my mother and Thomas, my two-year-old, to be able to visit the hospital at any time.
• Please note that I am a vegetarian.

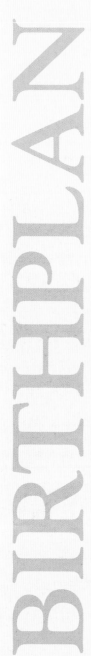

Name:

Doctor:

Midwife:

Birth attendant

Pain relief

Managing labor

Position for birth

Medical routines

The birth

Breastfeeding

Unforeseen problems

Notes

Useful addresses

LABOR AND BIRTH

American Academy of Husband-Coached Childbirth
P.O. Box 5224
Sherman Oaks, CA 91413
☎ 800–422–4784
www.bradleybirth.com

American Academy of Pediatrics
141 Northwest Point Blvd.
Elk Grove Village, IL
60007–1098
☎ 847–228–5005
www.aap.org

American College of Nurse Midwives (ACNM)
818 Connecticut Avenue, NW,
Suite 900
Washington, D.C. 20006
☎ 202–728–9860
www.acnm.org
Contact for midwife-assisted childbirth and prenatal care.

American College of Obstetricians and Gynecologists
409 12th Street, SW,
P.O. Box 96920
Washington, D.C. 20090–6920
www.acog.com

The Compassionate Friends
P.O. Box 3696
Oak Brook, IL 60522
☎ 630–990–0010
www.compassionatefriends.org
A national organization devoted to aiding parents who have experienced the death of a child.

Doulas of North America
1100 23rd Avenue E.
Seattle, WA 98112-3521
☎ 206–324–5440
www.dona.com
National resource for locating doulas.

Family Resource Coalition of America
20 North Wacher Drive,
Suite 1100
Chicago, IL 60606
☎ 312–341–0900
www.frca.org
Provides resources and information on family support.

Health Resources and Services Administration
Maternal and Child Health Bureau
Washington, D.C. 20201
☎ 301–443–0205
www.mchb.hrsa.gov
Federal agency providing programs for children and families.

International Childbirth Education Association (ICEA)
P.O. Box 20048
Minneapolis, MN 55420
☎ 800–624–4934
Nationwide organization dedicated to family-centered maternity care and freedom of choice in childbirth.

La Leche League International
1400 N. Meacham Road
Schaumburg, IL 60273–4048
☎ 847–519–7730
www.lalecheleague.com
Organization of women who offer practical support and advice for breastfeeding mothers.

Lamaze International
1200 19th Street, NW,
Suite 300
Washington, D.C. 20036–2422
☎ 800–368–4404
www.lamaze-childbirth.com
Devoted to the Lamaze method of childbirth.

National Association of Childbearing Centers (NACC)
3123 Gottschall Road
Perkiomenville, PA 18074
☎ 215–234–8068
www.birthcenters.org
Information about birth centers and childbearing alternatives.

National Center for Complementary and Alternative Medicine (NCCAM)
P.O. Box 8218
Silver Spring, MD 20907–8218
www.altmed.od.nih.gov
Provides information on alternative medicine and practitioners.

National Child Care Information Center
243 Church Street, NW,
2nd floor
Vienna, VA 22180
☎ 800–616–2242
www.nccic.org
Information and resources about daycare and related topics.

National Down's Syndrome Society
666 Broadway, 8th floor
New York, NY 10012-2317
☎ 800–221–4602
www.ndss.org

National Sudden Infant Death Syndrome Resource Center
2070 Chain Bridge Road,
Suite 450
Vienna, VA 22182
☎ 703–821–8955
www.circsol.com
Offers support to families who have lost babies and provides information about SIDS.

Parents Without Partners
401 North Michigan Avenue
Chicago, IL 60611–4267
☎ 312–644–6610
www.parentswithoutpartners.org
Provides information for single parents.

**Planned Parenthood Federation
of America, Inc.**
810 Seventh Avenue
New York, NY 10019
☎ 212–541–7800
www.plannedparenthood.org
*Offers a wide variety of reproductive
health services including tests for
pregnancy, prenatal care, and
infertility programs.*

SHARE
Pregnancy and Infant Loss
Support, Inc.
St. Joseph Health Center
300 First Capitol Drive
St. Charles, MO 63301–2893
☎ 314–947–6164
www.nationalshareoffice.com

**Spina Bifida Association of
America (SBAA)**
2590 McArthur Blvd., NW,
Suite 250
Washington, D.C. 20007–4226
☎ 800–621–3141
www.sbaa.org

Twin Services
Box 10066
Berkeley, CA 94709
☎ 501–524–0863

*Support and information for parents
of twins and multiples.*

United Cerebral Palsy
1660 L Street, NW, Suite 700
Washington, D.C. 20036
☎ 800–872–5827
www.upca.org
*Guidance and support for families
living with cerebral palsy.*

Further reading

Balaskas, Janet.
Active Birth,
Harvard Common Press, 1992.

Bradley, M.D., Robert A.
Husband-Coached Childbirth,
rev., Bantam, 1996.

Eisenberg, Arlene, Hathaway, Sandee E., and Murkoff, Heidi E.
What to Expect When You're Expecting,
rev., Simon & Schuster, 1996.

Fazal, Anwar and La Leche League.
The Womanly Art of Breastfeeding,
rev., La Leche League, 1997.

Green, Dr. Christopher.
Dr. Green's Baby Book,
Ballantine Books, 1998.

Kitzinger, Sheila.
Breastfeeding Your Baby,
rev., Knopf, 1998.

Kitzinger, Sheila.
The Complete Book of Pregnancy and Childbirth,
rev., Knopf, 1996.

Klein, Alan H., and Ganon, Jill Alison.
Caring for Your Premature Baby,
Harper, 1998.

Korte, Diana, and Scaer, Roberta.
A Good Birth, A Safe Birth,
Harvard Common Press, 1992.

Leach, Penelope.
Your Baby and Child,
rev., Knopf, 1997.

Malmstrom, Patricia, and Poland, Janet.
The Art of Parenting Twins,
Ballantine Books, 1999.

Spencer, Paula, with The Editors of Parenting Magazine.
Parenting Guide to Pregnancy & Childbirth,
Ballantine Books, 1998.

Spock, Dr. Benjamin, and Parker, Stephen J.
Dr. Spock's Baby and Child Care,
rev., Pocket Books, 1998.

Wilen, Joan.
The Perfect Name for the Perfect Baby,
rev., Ballantine Books, 1997.

Index